Stuttering:
From Theory to Practice

Edited by
Margaret Fawcus

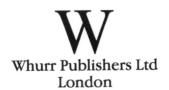

Whurr Publishers Ltd
London

© 1995 Whurr Publishers Ltd
Whurr Publishers Ltd
19b Compton Terrace, London N1 2UN, England
Reprinted 1998

British Library Cataloguing in Publication Data
A catalogue record for this book is available from the
British Library.

ISBN 1-897635-81-8

Photoset by Stephen Cary
Printed and bound in the UK by Athenaeum Press Ltd,
Gateshead, Tyne & Wear

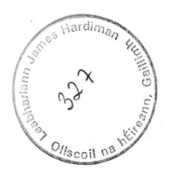

Contents

Introduction

Over the past two decades we have seen the emergence of an essentially British school of speech and language therapy for children and adults with disfluency disorders. It is an eclectic approach, recognising that programmes of therapy can seldom meet all the individual needs of most people who stutter. It has taken on board much of what is the best of American ideas on intervention, but has tended to avoid the strong dichotomy between the speak-more-fluently and the stutter-more-fluently schools of thought. It is perhaps the profound influence of Kelly and his development of the personal construct view of personality that has led British therapists to place much less emphasis on fluency techniques than previously. Bitter experience, for both client and therapist, has shown that such fluency gains are a fragile framework on which to base lasting change.

It is a sad reflection on the current state of the National Health Service in Britain that we are failing to meet the needs of many people who stutter, despite the increasing expertise, and indeed confidence, which have been developing over the past few years. If there is one good thing to come of the present restriction on the provision of speech therapy, it is the emergence of an increasingly effective lobby by The Association of Stammerers themselves.

This book attempts to encompass most of the essential issues surrounding stuttering — including the development of stuttering, the psychology of the stutterer and approaches to intervention. It reflects on many of the current issues facing clinicians and attempts to present a cohesive picture of the state of the art from the essentially personal standpoint of a group of speech and language therapists who share the same philosophy. The chapters bear testimony to the creativity that a personal construct approach seems to engender.

The final chapter looks at stuttering and speech and language therapy from the perspective of the stutterer himself. It also outlines the work of the Association for Stammerers (the British counterpart of the Speak Easy Foundation and the National Stuttering Project in the USA). Whilst the word stuttering is otherwise used throughout this book, the word stammering is normally used in the United Kingdom.

We hope that this book will succeed in giving some idea of the creativity which can be generated within this theoretical and philosophical framework.

Margaret Fawcus, February 1995

Chapter 1
The Development of Stuttering: Implications for Early Intervention

MARGARET FAWCUS

Whilst the development of high technology may one day discover a single, neat cause of stuttering, the majority of therapists now subscribe to what might be described as an interactional model of aetiology. It is recognised that there are a number of predisposing, precipitating and maintaining factors which determine whether a particular child will develop a temporary or chronic problem of disfluency. People who stutter are a heterogeneous rather than a homogenous group, which has complex implications for intervention programmes.

There has been relatively little research into the development of stuttering. There are at least two reasons for this: in the first place, research is bedevilled by the number of variables involved. Taking into account the physiological, psycholinguistic and psychosocial factors involved, Rommel *et al.* (1993) estimated that about 300 variables are relevant to the onset of stuttering. This makes research into this area a formidable task. In the second place, most of the information available on the phenomenon of early stuttering relies on the retrospective reports of parents, which may or may not have been accurately observed or recalled. Despite these problems, there is increasing interest in the very early development of stuttering. Yairi and Lewis (1984) made a study of 10 two- and three-year-olds who were diagnosed as stuttering and who were referred within two months of onset. This provided a unique opportunity to study these early disfluencies. It was found that the experimental group were three times as non-fluent as the control group. Despite a degree of overlap, and large variability within each group, stutterers and non-stutterers 'emerged as representing two fairly distinctive population samples'.

Early Stuttering or Normal Non-fluency?

There has been considerable recent focus on the need to make a differential diagnosis between the disfluencies observable in the speech of the majority of children at some time or other and the non-fluencies exhibited by children diagnosed as stuttering. Are they quantitatively and qualitatively the same? This has, in fact, been one of the great debates of recent times.

It would obviously be useful if children at risk of developing chronic stuttering could be identified as a group. Yairi and Lewis (1984) found some significant differences between the two groups. The experimental group demonstrated more repetition units on disfluent words, and their speech was characterised by sound prolongations and part-word repetitions.

Pindzola's Protocol for Differentiating the Incipient Stutterer (1987) is based on the notion that stuttering can be distinguished from normal non-fluencies. Depending on the type of non-fluency and the frequency of occurrence, judgements are made on a three-point scale: probably normal, questionable and probably abnormal. Interjections are regarded as probably normal, with repetitions and prolongations classified as questionable or probably abnormal. The use of an intrusive 'schwa' vowel is also regarded as an indication that the the child is stuttering, along with any sign of visible struggle.

Traditionally, stuttering was said to develop from effortless repetitions of syllables or words, with no apparent awareness on the child's part or evidence of struggle behaviour. Clinical experience, however, suggests that this is not always the case and the present author has seen signs of awareness and tension in children as young as 2;6 years, with no sense of a gradual onset.

There has been a considerable shift from Johnson's (1959) view that normal non-fluencies and early stuttering are one and the same thing, and that stuttering begins to emerge as a problem only when these non-fluencies are focused and commented upon by parents who perceive them as abnormal. In other words, it is only when the non-fluencies become the object of 'social penalty' that the child starts to be aware that there is something 'wrong' with his speech, and the stage is set for the possible development of a chronic problem.

In his continuity hypothesis, Bloodstein (1970) took a closer look at Johnson's data, and began to formulate a more comprehensive and complex view of the origins of stuttering behaviour. Looking at part-word repetitions, for example, he found that the most severe stutterer had over three units of repetition, with one non-stutterer having two units of repetition. Whilst it was clear that the stuttering group had more units of repetition, there was no sharp dichotomy between the two groups. Moreover, he concluded that there was a consistency effect in the distribution of these part-word repetitions for both the control and the experimental group. Bloodstein quoted a study by Egland (1938) who looked at the part-word repetitions in 26 non-stutterers (aged 5–6 years) and 3 stutterers (aged 3–4 years).

Non-fluencies had a similar distribution in both groups, occurring at the beginning of words and sentences and on unfamiliar polysyllabic words. Syllable repetitions tended to occur in both groups when asking questions. Bloodstein found that prolongations occurred in 80% of stutterers and 30% of non-stutterers.

Bloodstein came to the conclusion that each of the features of disfluent speech occurs in readily discernible amounts in both groups, but more frequently in young stutterers than nonstutterers. He therefore felt it reasonable to hypothesise that there is a basic continuity between the forms of behaviour generally identified as early stuttering and at least some of the features of early normal non-fluencies.

Surprisingly, this also included evidence of some forcing behaviour, which one might reasonably have supposed would be found only in the experimental group. He also reported on struggle behaviour as early as 2 years, and a number of the control group parents said that their children seemed aware that they were not speaking normally on occasions.

These findings suggest that some young children are sufficiently disfluent to be aware that they are experiencing difficulty and, furthermore, that they are already beginning to try and force words out. This takes us beyond the idea that early stuttering always develops from effortless non-fluencies which are erroneously labelled as stuttering by concerned parents. None the less, we cannot underestimate Johnson's contribution in alerting us to the role of parents and other carers who often unwittingly contribute to the development of stuttering.

Whilst assessment procedures are important in trying to establish whether a child is exhibiting normal non-fluencies or early stuttering, there is a very real danger that other important variables may not receive the attention they merit in the search for objective measures. In addition, the cut-off point between normal non-fluencies and early stuttering is essentially rather an arbitrary one. It is clear that we need continuing longitudinal studies.

The Vulnerability of the Child

Emotional Vulnerability

There is no doubt that some children are more vulnerable than others, both physically and emotionally. This vulnerability is probably the most important variable to be considered in both the development of stuttering and in the management of the child who stutters. Bloodstein *et al.* (1965) spoke of the child who is insecure, has an excessive need for approval, is dependent and fearful and has a low tolerance level for frustration. Such a child, they suggest, is particularly vulnerable to environmental pressures and is 'especially quick to accept a concept of himself as a failure'.

Whilst Wendell Johnson placed considerable emphasis on the role of the parent in his semantogenic theory of stuttering, he wrote of a trilogy of perceptual awareness: the parents' awareness of the child's non-fluencies, the child's awareness of his own non-fluencies and his awareness of the parental reaction to these non-fluencies. In advocating an indirect approach in the management of early stuttering and working only through the parents, clinicians have in the past not always taken sufficient account of the child's awareness of his own disfluent speech.

In formulating a more global view of the onset of stuttering, Bloodstein suggested that most children experience minor tensions and fragmentations in their speech. In some cases, communicative failure related to articulatory or linguistic problems may be so severe and frequent that 'the child may develop a more or less chronic belief in the difficulty of speech' which gradually develops into 'identifiable episodes of stuttering'.

This, of course, has important implications for intervention, because not only are we dealing with environmental factors which may hinder communication and foster the development of non-fluency, but we must also tread a careful path through the child's own feelings about his speech and how others react to it.

We must not underestimate how quickly a child may begin to perceive himself as a failure. This will be dependent on a number of factors, including the child's sensitivity to criticism and reprimand. Some children are emotionally much 'tougher' than others and seem oblivious or uncaring about quite high levels of social penalty. Other children are very aware of and sensitive to quite subtle signs of parental anxiety or disapproval. Unfortunately, the child is frequently hampered by his lack of linguistic concepts to express his anxiety or to seek reassurance.

Physical Vulnerability

Johnson's (1959) study, in which he looked at 150 children who stuttered and 150 non-stutterers (age range 2–8 years) found no significant differences in the physical development of the two groups. This included such speech milestones as first word and first use of sentences. However, Andrews and Harris (1964) found that poor and delayed speech was clearly associated with stuttering. The stuttering group were some four months retarded in the acquisition of first phrases, and more of them had articulatory defects than the control group. If we add the variable of a positive family history, we have a group who are five times more 'at risk' of developing a stutter than those children without these factors. In an earlier study by Morley (1957) similar findings were reported: as a group, the stutterers were some three months delayed in the production of their first word, five months delayed in the use of first phrases, and nearly a year delayed in the acquisition of intelligible speech.

Yairi (1993) cited a study by Louko *et al.* (1990) in which children who stuttered had more phonological problems than their non-stuttering peers. St Louis *et al.* (1991) also found that a substantial proportion of school-aged stutterers manifested coexisting communication disorders, notably in the realms of articulation and voice. In the first 15 months of a multifactorial longitudinal study, Rommel *et al.* (1993) also reported that almost 60% of 41 pre-school children examined presented with articulatory problems in addition to stuttering. In the majority of cases, these problems were not very severe.

Whilst many children who stutter present with normal linguistic development at the phonological, semantic and syntactical levels, recent research does seem to show that a significant number have phonological problems in particular. One possible hypothesis is that there is a delayed neurological maturation which makes the child vulnerable to both fluency and articulation problems (I am using the term articulation to include both articulatory and phonological disorders). This would tend to suggest some form of motor deficit, although the fact that many, indeed most, children who stutter also have periods when they are fluent would tend to argue against this. It may be, however, that the presence of disfluencies occurs only when there are additional stress factors present which overload the system; for example, an 'at risk' child who is exposed to an environment where her speech models have a rapid rate of utterance.

In a study of speech rates in children with a mean age of 4 years and 10 years (Fawcus, 1973) it was found that their speech was significantly slower than that of adult speakers. The children were given repetition tasks and in spontaneous speech pauses were deleted so that the 'absolute rate of articulation' (Goldmann-Eisler, 1968) could be calculated. Such a finding suggests that pre-school children are growing up in an environment with adult speech rates which they are unable to match, and which may therefore provide stressful speech models. Even more important was the finding which showed that the rate of articulation of boys (at both 4 and 10 years of age) was significantly slower than the girls in the study, which may be one explanation for the gender differences in stuttering. Meyers and Freeman (1985) found that mothers of stutterers talked significantly faster than mothers of non-stutterers. However, they also found that the mothers of non-stutterers also spoke more rapidly to children who stuttered. They came to the conclusion that it was difficult to determine whether the child stuttered because the parent had a rapid rate of utterance, or whether the mother spoke more quickly because of the child's stuttering and slower rate of speech. They suggest that both may be true and 'the effect is both interactive and circular'.

Van Riper (1972) suggested that when a person stuttered on a word there was a 'temporal disruption of the simultaneous and successive programming of muscular movements required to produce speech'. He went on to conclude that temporal disruption is the core behaviour of stuttering. As Van Riper said, speech requires precisely timed motor sequences, and the normal distribution of motor ability would produce some individuals who have difficulty in accomplishing that timimg. He put forward the idea that the 1% who stutter 'represent the extreme end of the normal distribution in co-ordinative ability or stress vulnerability'. Van Riper's theory is an appealing one, as it can accommodate fluency as well as disfluency in the speech of the stutterer. He suggests that the stress of some speech situations adds to the stress of an already over-burdened timing system. Young children are much more vulnerable to fluency disruption because their motor skills are less stable. Van Riper sees early prolongations and repetitions as the natural consequence of mistiming. Individual differences in the older child or adult can be explained by their response to the experience of 'broken' speech and the anxiety this can generate.

More recent research points to the possibility that slow voice onset time and voice reaction time may be causal factors in stuttering. Perkins (1986) concludes that 'the most incontrovertible lead, cast in broadest terms, is that stuttering is a discoordination of muscular and/or aerody-namic coordinations among the phonatory, articulatory, and possibly respiratory system'. It might equally well be argued, however, that slow voice onset time is a result of stuttering. It is not within the scope of this chapter to detail or discuss recent research into the physiology of stut-tering, but we must be alert to future implications for management.

Speech is a complex amd rapid motor skill. The adult speaker produces in the region of five syllables a second (Fawcus, 1973) with the coordination of some 100 muscles (Lenneberg, 1967) in the production of breath flow, voicing and articulation. We know that the development of the child's phonemic repertoire is linked to the 'ease' of production of speech sounds (Locke, 1972). If we looked at the development of stut-tering in terms of skill acquisition, then the fact that speech can be disrupted should come as no surprise. What is surprising, perhaps, is the fact that motor skill acquisition has not received the attention it deserves in studies of speech development (a penalty, perhaps, of our fascination with phonology at the expense of articulation!) .

Genetics and Gender

One fact which is not in dispute is that stuttering runs in families, but there has been much less agreement about whether stuttering is inher-ited and, if so, exactly what is inherited.

Johnson (1959) found that 23% of both experimental group mothers and fathers in his study had a positive family history, against 5% and 6% of control group mothers and fathers respectively. Andrews and Harris (1964) found that 38% of the children in their study had a family history of stuttering.

It is therefore not surprising that the notion has been put forward that many cases of stuttering have a genetic basis that interacts with environmental forces (Yairi, 1993). Ambrose *et al.* (1993) consider that there is now significant statistical evidence for a major genetic locus for stuttering. The question remains, however: what precisely is inherited?

In view of findings which suggest that stutterers have a history of poor and late talking (Andrews and Harris, 1964) and other researchers having found a significant increase in articulatory problems (Louko *et al.*, 1990; Rommel *et al.*, 1993 ; St Louis *et al.*, 1991) we might postulate that children inherit some kind of genetic blueprint, either in the form of delayed neurological maturation or a motor deficit. Both Yairi (1993) and Andrews and Harris (1964) have spoken of a 'genetic loading'. Yairi went on to suggest that a child who recovers from stuttering may have a genetically milder form of susceptibility than those who become chronic stutterers.

One other accepted fact is that there is a gender factor in stuttering. Whilst the ratio of males to females is not so great in children as it is in the adult population, ratios of 2:1 (Yairi, 1993) and 3:1 (Rommel et al., 1993) have been reported. We find that other communication problems are more prevalent in boys, who also tend to be later than girls in developing speech (Robinson, 1987). These facts would tend to support both a genetic factor and the possibility of a slower pattern of physical maturation. This is perhaps the genetic matrix of which Andrews and Harris (1964) wrote. The fact that boys tend to speak more slowly than girls, as already mentioned (Fawcus, 1973) may also point in the same direction. This cluster of findings suggests that boys are more vulnerable to fluency disruption during the crucial period of speech development.

Before leaving the question of gender, one other interesting fact has emerged from Yairi's (1993) study: girls seem to develop stuttering at an earlier age than boys, and this may be because they are earlier in speech development and are therefore reaching the vulnerable stage of putting words together at an earlier age Whilst Johnson (1959) put the age of onset of stuttering between 3;6 and 4 years, Yairi and Ambrose (1992) estimated that 68% of all onsets occurred between 25 and 41 months. They comment that the lower age of onset now seen is closer to important events in speech and language development, and should encourage research into the relationship between stuttering and physiological and neuroanatomical maturation processes underlying these events.

The fact that the male:female ratio is considerably higher in adults (Yairi, op. cit.) suggests that females are more likely to 'grow out of stammering', which may be linked to their greater linguistic competence in the early years.

Linguistic Factors

It would seem that the appearance of non-fluencies, whether normal or abnormal, coincides with the child's emerging syntax and an increasing use of language to communicate his needs and feelings and to respond to the speech of others in his environment. Starkweather (1987) stated that 'increased syntactic, semantic, phonologic and pragmatic knowledge all contribute to the demand for fluency...this increased syntactic knowledge is a demand on motor speech production'. The young child is not only acquiring the complex motor skills of speech, but is also coming to grips with syntactic rules and searching for the vocabulary required but not always possessed.

The articulatory and phonological difficulties which are found in association with stuttering in young children have already been discussed. What about their semantic and syntactic development? Research in this area is conflicting and may reflect the particular sample of young stutterers investigated, as it is clear that they are not a homogenous group. There does seem to be a group of children (Van Riper's Track II) who do present with speech and language delay, whilst other children who stutter have followed a normal developmental path.

Wall (1980) made a comparative study of syntax in a small group of four male stutterers (aged 5;6–6;6) matched for age, sex, parental occupation and birth order with a group of four non-stutterers. The results suggested that the children who stuttered used 'simpler, less mature language' than the non-stutterers. A study by Kadi-Hairifi and Howell (1992) looked at syntax in the spontaneous speech of a group of 17 subjects between the ages of 2;7 and 12;6 years, matched with a group of fluent controls. They found no evidence that the experimental group used less developed syntax than their controls. The mean length of utterance of the children who stuttered was in line with normal language development. In the preliminary findings of their five-year longitudinal study, Rommel *et al.* (1993) reported that there was no evidence of what they call a general language delay in 41 subjects.

One of the most recently reported studies (Weiss and Zebrowski, 1994) looked at the narrative ability of eight children who stuttered matched for age and gender with a fluent control group. The young stutterers did not perform significantly differently from the non-stutterers on most of the narrative measures used. In both re-telling a story and creating original stories, the non-fluent children were as grammatically competent as their fluent peers and conveyed the same amount of information. They reported, however, that there were some subtle differences which could be related to stuttering. In re-telling a story to 'naive' listeners, for example, the stuttering group produced shorter and less elaborated accounts. The authors suggested that an awareness of their stuttering and a desire to avoid it, rather than a lack of competence, could account for this difference. The stories they created tended to be shorter, with fewer completed episodes.

The study by Klein and Rustin (1991) suggested that language difficulties may persist into adolescence (see Chapter 5).

From the studies cited above, it does seem clear that a significant proportion of children who stutter are also at risk of associated speech and language problems. Such findings have important implications for the assessment, intervention and possible educational attainment of children who are referred for therapy.

Considerations for Education

There seems to be very little information on the educational status of the child who stutters, although clinical experience would suggest that attainment may be affected because of both emotional and linguistic factors.

In their study of 86 nine- to 11-year-old stutterers, Andrews and Harris (1964) looked at the reading skills of 80 of their subjects, comparing their performance with 80 non-stuttering peers. They used Schonell's (1950) tests of word recognition and word comprehension. The experimental group achieved slightly lower reading quotients on both tasks, but the differences were not statistically different. Using the Wechsler Intelligence Scale for Children (1949) they found that the stuttering group had a mean IQ of 95 compared with a mean IQ of 102 for the control group. This result was statistically significant, and might have explained the tendency towards poorer performance on reading tasks.

A study by McDowell (1928) quoted by Nippold and Schwarz (1990) examined the reading ability of 45 stutterers and 45 non-stutterers, matched for chronological age, intelligence, gender, native language and racial background. Both groups had a mean IQ of 103, and the average chronological age of each was approximately 10 years. Although the mean scores of the stuttering group were lower than the control group (on word, sentence and paragraph meaning, arithmetic and spelling) these results did not reach statistical significance. Daly (1981), also quoted by Nippold and Schwarz, looked at the reading ability of 138 stutterers, with an age range of 8;1 to 20;0 years. He was interested in studying the performance of sub-groups of stutterers, and successfully assigned 83% of the subjects to one of Van Riper's tracks. Of the 33 stutterers assigned to Track II, 32 had a history of delayed speech and language development, and 13 of these (39%) had also had reading difficulties.

As Nippold and Schwarz (1990) claim, research involving non-stutterers has shown that poor readers often have a history of delayed speech development, exhibiting a greater frequency of phonological, morphological, syntactic and semantic deficits than their peer group who learn to read with no apparent difficulty. They go on to say it is possible that stutterers having a history of delayed language onset may be more vulnerable to reading problems than those who develop langauage normally. It has been suggested (Williams *et al.*, 1969, in Nippold and Schwarz, 1990) that academic delays in stutterers might be caused by poor participation in classroom activities, compounded by teachers' reluctance to demand such participation.

We know remarkably little about general academic achievement in school-age stutterers. Here again, clinical experience suggests that there is frequently poorer performance than normal in reading, handwriting and spelling. These are subjective impressions, however, which need further investigation. Positively, Nippold and Schwarz (1990) recommend that 'steps could be taken to to restructure a stutterer's learning environment so that classroom participation is maximised in ways that avoid embarrassment and loss of self-esteem'.

An important study of school-age stutterers from a teacher's perspective has been carried out by Frewer (1993). Frewer states that 'many children who stutter face significant difficulties in school not experienced by their fluent peers'. She considers that the introduction of the National Curriculum into British schools, with its greater emphasis on oral skills, is likely to increase these difficulties.

Of the 12 secondary school children in her study (11–18 years) all but one felt that their stammer affected them in school to some extent. Six pupils specifically mentioned their reluctance to ask questions and seek help, and 11 referred to in-class avoidance of verbal interaction. A number of children absented themselves from lessons because of the speaking activities involved. Eleven of the stutterers had experienced teasing or bullying which occurred as a result of their speech handicap.

Of the 37 teachers who participated in the study, over 50% had contact with a child who stuttered at the time of the survey. Only one teacher had received any information about stuttering, though 84% of the teachers would have welcomed information or training on the management of children who stutter in the classroom. Frewer concluded that more information should be available for teachers and counselling should be available for all pupils. She also concluded that there is a need for further research in the relationship between stuttering and academic achievement.

Grove and Walton (1981) found that teachers with a greater knowledge of stuttering showed more desirable attitudes to stutterers, which lends support to Frewer's recommendation that more information on stuttering should be made available to teachers. Lass *et al.* (1992) also found a strong relationship between teachers' knowledge and attitudes, and suggested that as the teacher is such a significant person in a child's life, the problem of avoiding negative stereotypes of children who stutter should be addressed in teacher training and continuing education.

One might reasonably expect anxiety and loss of self-esteem to lead to academic under-achievement, quite apart from the child's unwillingness to participate in verbal activities. School is a critical time in the development of a child's self-image and yet we know very little about the effect of stuttering on the child's academic attainment or self-esteem.

The Role of Parents and Peers

In discussing the parental role in the development of stuttering we must also take into account the contribution of any significant others in the child's environment. In fact, we know very little about the parent group as a whole, apart from the studies by Johnson (1959) and Andrews and Harris (1964). Whilst Johnson found the experimental and control groups of parents to be essentially more alike than different, there was a tendency for the experimental group parents, particularly the mothers, to show less satisfaction with their children, their spouses and their circumstances than the control group parents. They tended to operate with more demanding expectations and anxiety, and rated their children less favourably in terms of social development. This extended to their children's speech development, which some regarded as much slower than average though this was not borne out by the facts. Johnson found that the experimental group of children had been subjected to more pressures in various aspects of training. It was these findings, and the belief that these same parents viewed their children's normal non-fluencies as stuttering, that led to his diagnosogenic or semantic theory of the onset of stuttering. The parent was held to have a central role in the child's gradually increasing awareness that there was something wrong with his speech.

Andrews and Harris (1964) looked at the parents of their 86 nine- to 11-year-olds and found a rather different picture. In the first place, there was a degree of 'social deprivation' in the home, and they commented that a higher proportion of mothers in the experimental group had a poor ability to manage. These findings were presumably regarded as reponsible for the adverse environmental factors which acted on the 'genetic matrix' to produce stuttering. They commented that the mothers of stutterers demonstrated a tendency to fail to cope in providing an adequate home environment for their children.

In their component model of stuttering, Riley and Riley (1979) list three interpersonal components: a disruptive communicative environment, unrealistic parental expectations and an abnormal parental need for their child to stutter. Of the 54 children in their study, 53% were reported by parents to be subject to disrupted communication attempts, including interruptions and creating a speaking environment in which the child had insufficient time to organise his thoughts. Some 51% of parents had unrealistic expectations of their children. They went on to say that 'competition was a strong factor within the family constellation. Parents verbally or attitudinally demanded perfection from their child academically, behaviourally and developmentally.' These findings would certainly accord with those of Johnson.

Starkweather (1987) has also written of the demands made by the child's environment which may exceed his capacity to cope with these demands. He mentions rapid rate of utterance and rapid turn-taking which inadvertently place a demand on the child to talk rapidly. In addition, the parents may create a sense of urgency and rush, which will place further demands on the child to get his message over quickly. His demands and capacities model is discussed more fully in Chapter 3.

Competition may also come from siblings, particularly if they are verbally more competent and tend to monopolise the conversation. It can be difficult to find 'speaking time' in a talkative family.

Bloodstein (1958) also suggested that a child who has spoken unusually early or well can, in a subtle way, create an atmosphere of heightened expectation with regard to speech. In addition to the child's own awareness of the 'imperfections' in her speech (such as articulation errors or non-fluencies), she 'must be assisted to regard them as failures or difficulties by a cooperative environment. An important source of the stutterer's belief in the difficulty of speech are the anxieties and demands focused by parents with varying degrees of subtlety on the communication process.'

Having discussed the part played by parents and significant others in the development of stuttering, we must now consider what effect these influences have on children's reactions to their early non-fluencies.

Every case is unique in the way that linguistic, psychosocial and environmental factors operate and interact to create the problem of chronic stuttering. It now seems clear that children may be aware of tensions and fragmentations in their speech at a very early age, and with this growing awareness we begin to see the development of behaviours which are designed to try and get words out. This awareness may arise out of the frustration the child is experiencing in trying to get his message across. As time goes on, however, he also begins to realise that he has an unacceptable speech problem to be avoided, hidden, disguised or postponed. Van Riper and Bloodstein have described the typical processes that occur in their tracks and phases, but we lack detailed accounts of the behaviours and the time-scale involved in individual children.

If we accept that there may be some neurogenic factor operating in the early repetitions and prolongations which signal the onset of stuttering, the complex of behaviours which cluster together to create each individual stutter are almost certainly learned reactions to these early fragmentations. They may arise from ill-informed advice, such as 'take a deep breath' which results in a habitual inspiratory gasp. The attempt on the feared word may be postponed by the use of repeated interjections, or the child may try and take a running jump at the word by back-tracking ('My name is...my name is...my name is...'). A 10-year-old tried to hide his stutter by putting his hand over his mouth and pretending to yawn which led to a very abnormal habitual behaviour. Almost inevitably, increased tension is used to try and get the word out, but this only serves to make normal speech production impossible.

Early Intervention

Whilst current research may point in the direction of some physiological factor in early stuttering, it is clear that the natural history of stuttering involves many other possible variables. It is as if there is a pattern of interwoven threads, possibly unique in more or less subtle ways for each child. The therapist's role is to try and tease out these different threads and then to try and evaluate the relative weighting to give to each one. Sometimes a thread seems to stand out with particular clarity and may, above all, be the cause of the non-fluency. A three-year-old, the only son of Polish parents, was referred to the author. It emerged that the child was coping with English at his nursery school and Polish at home. The parents admitted that he became very upset when they spoke in front of and to him in Polish. Their wish that he should grow up to speak Polish was understandable but it was suggested that in view of his distress it would be advisable to speak only in English for the time being. They accepted this advice and the problem resolved itself. This was an unusually clear example of a single thread that appeared to be reponsible for the child's non-fluency although parental anxiety probably also played a part.

The case quoted above is a very neat example of the demands and capacities model (Starkweather, 1987) where the young child, negotiating the motor and linguistic complexities of the spoken word, was unable to cope with the very understandable demands the parents were placing on him. The parents were caring and concerned, and anxious that their only son should learn their mother tongue. Both parents and child had their different needs in terms of therapeutic intervention. It was essential, if such intervention was to be effective, that the situation be handled with an understanding of a dual dilemma.

Can Stuttering be Prevented?

One of the many great debates on the causes and management of stuttering has focused on the notion of prevention. If we accept the importance of the parents' role in the development of stuttering, it should be possible to educate/counsel parents in ways of handling the early non-fluencies, which may well be regarded as a phenomenon present in the speech of the majority of young children. However, Hamre (1992) has challenged the belief that stuttering can be prevented. He maintains that parents can readily distinguish between stuttering and normal disfluency, and by the time they seek help the time to prevent stuttering has long since passed. He recommends that a treatment construct should replace the prevention construct in the management of early childhood stuttering. Nevertheless, the majority of therapists would maintain that there are cases where parents and significant others in the child's environment are reacting with undue anxiety to normal disfluencies. We are dealing with a wide spectrum of parents, some of whom are particularly ready to perceive problems in their children. There is also the 'perceptual orientation' of parents who themselves stutter or who have close relatives who stutter. This must surely colour their perceptions of any disfluent patterns of speech.

In many cases, however, Hamre will be right because the child has not been referred at a stage where parental counselling might have been effective. By this time, the child himself has probably become part of the equation. Whilst Johnson's famous dictum that stuttering begins in the ear of the listener and not in the mouth of the child had a justifiably important influence on the management of young stutterers, it seemed to ignore the child's own awareness of his disfluencies. Unfortunately, the indirect approach to the treatment of early stuttering, which Johnson's ideas tended to foster, ignored the fact that children can become aware of their difficulties at a very early stage in the development of stuttering.

A boy of 2;6 years, known to the author, had already begun to show signs of struggle behaviour and would put his hand in front of his mouth when he blocked. Happily, thoughtful intervention by caring parents gave him the reasurrance he needed, and the stutter did not develop into a chronic problem. An intelligent six-year-old had already developed a strategy of spelling out the words he could not say. With reactions of this order to tensions and fragmentations in their speech, we clearly cannot afford to leave the child out of the intervention process, unless we are very sure that he is unaware of his disfluencies or other communication failures.

A number of possible scenarios seem to emerge: we have a child who is sensitively aware of his failure to make himself understood or of his difficulty in getting words out. He is equally sensitive to his parents' reactions to his speech, even though these may be non-verbal and barely perceptible. He is potentially at risk of developing low self-esteem as well as increasing anxiety about the tensions and fragmentations in his speech. Here the therapist will be particularly concerned with the child himself, building up his self-esteem and increasing his confidence in his ability to communicate. This child is very vulnerable to fluency disrupters and to social penalties that he may begin to encounter.

On the other hand, we may have a child who has a much higher tolerance level, who is more confident and outgoing. His speech development may have proceeded normally and he may have experienced no difficulty in making himself understood. He is, however, in a competitive speech environment, with older siblings competing for speaking time and parents who speak rapidly and have a hectic lifestyle. At three years he is still struggling to master the motor and linguistic skills of speech and cannot cope with the demands of his particular speech environment. It is hardly surprising that his fluency breaks down as he tries to match the speed of his parents' speech and to break into family conversations. Here the management would tend to centre on the environmental factors, with the idea of creating a more speaker-friendly environment. The aim would be to encourage a more listening environment in which the child can find time to talk.

In other cases we may feel that the weighting is more equally balanced between the child himself and his environment.

The relative weighting in any case must be based on careful observation of the child and his speech and his relationships with the family and other children. Even more important are the insights we may gain by talking with the parents in an empathic and non-judgemental manner – even when the temptation is to be disapproving and directive!

Parents can become angry and defensive, and understandably distressed, by a failure to appreciate that they are human and may therefore be impatient and irritable when they are tired or when the children are particularly trying. In most cases they act in the best interests of their children, but may not know how to deal with the situation. Undoubtedly, being an imperfect parent has helped me to appreciate the parents' point of view. We must make the parents feel secure about their parenting by reinforcing what they do well and by helping them to achieve insights into where they are going wrong without stirring up guilt and resentment.

It may require considerable tact and skill on the therapist's part to discover the various factors which are operating within the family and which may be affecting the child who stutters. It will also require insight and honesty on the parents' part in being prepared to discuss the problem as they see it. It is essential that the therapist is a credulous and non-judgemental listener, who has an understanding of the pressures the parents are coping with at home. An empathy with them is as important as an empathy with the child. The words we use are, to quote Lenny Henry, "crucial" and we must make sensitive and careful use of them in our sessions with both the child and the parents.

The suggestions we make to parents should be positive and realistic. The following information sheet attempts to increase the parents' understanding of the problem as well as suggesting ways in which they might help their child.

How to Help your Child

Learn to listen: this is not always easy when there are so many things competing for your attention. Give your child time to talk and make sure that you are really listening. If this is just not possible at that particular moment, then explain why and promise that you will listen later. Talking with your child helps him develop language and learn about conversation,which in turn helps to give him confidence in speaking.

If your child stutters, give him the time he needs to speak and be patient and reassuring if he seems distressed. How to react in the most helpful way will depend to some extent on the age of your child and the way he stammers, so seek the advice of your speech and language therapist if you are not sure what to do.

Provide a helpful speech model: a young child's rate of speech is slower than that of an adult – in the first place, he is having to negotiate the complexities of finding the words he wants and putting them together into sentences. He does not always possess the vocabulary he needs or an understanding of the rules which govern sentence production. Second, he is developing the motor skills of a very rapid and complex activity in which he has to control and coordinate the muscles of breathing, voice production and articulation. He cannot match the rate at which adults speak, and an environment where adults speak quickly and use long, complicated sentences may add to the child's difficulties. So try and speak a little more slowly, and use simpler sentences which provide your child with an easier speech model to copy.

Avoid making demands on your child's speech – this is particularly important when your child is tired, distressed or unwell. We often bombard children with questions when they come home from school, at a low physical and sometimes emotional ebb. Save your curiosity until they have had time to eat and unwind. Performing in front of relatives or friends can be stressful and should be avoided unless your child enjoys that sort of attention!

Aim for consistency in setting out behavioural guidelines – this is one of the hardest goals to achieve. The way we are feeling as parents so often determines how we react to our childrens' behaviour. Something which we can tolerate when we are on top of things can be a source of extreme irritation when we are tired and harrassed! Try and set out clear, sensible and realistic guidelines for the behaviour you expect (the House Rules, if you like). Try not to be too rigid about issues of cleanliness, eating habits or perfect speech. We all want our children to be paragons of virtue, but we have to temper these ambitions with an understanding of the childrens' own need to be accepted as they are. This may include not doing very well at school because they find the work difficult and not because they are lazy.

Try and avoid discussing difficult and fraught issues when you are short of time and patience, or when everyone is tired. Try and make yourself approachable so that children are not frightened to come and talk about their worries.

Be prepared to apologise to your child if you feel you have acted unreasonably or been unduly harsh. It is important that adults can admit to being wrong if we expect our children to be equally honest. At the same time, children need to realise that parents have their needs (like some time to themselves and some help in the house) and their problems (like having to cope with a job, and then coming home to cooking, washing and cleaning). It is not always easy to be fair and reasonable when you are feeling tired, and this should be explained as soon as children are old enough to understand.

Dealing with bad behaviour: there are no easy answers to many of our childrens' behaviour problems. Because we are often emotionally involved with our children we are not always the best person to deal with them, and may need to seek help from experienced professionals. Bad behaviour is often an expression of anxieties and conflicts that young children may not be able to put into words because they do not yet have the 'language' of feelings and emotions. Sometimes we can guess what is wrong and give them the explanation and reassurance they need. Remember that bad behaviours are often inconvenient behaviours, like children playing football and getting their clothes dirty when you have just washed and ironed them! Getting over-tired is a very common cause of difficult behaviour, so make sure your child is getting the rest he needs.

Children do need the security of clearly spelled-out boundaries, and it is difficult for them to cope with inconsistent rules of behaviour. It is not possible to reason with very young children, and sometimes the best way of dealing with temper tantrums and such like is a period of time out, before you lose your temper!

Children use up a great deal of energy in growing, playing and learning. They cannot really benefit from school if they are watching television until late at night, or if they never have quiet times in which to unwind.

If your children are secure in the knowledge that you love and care about them, and are interested in their achievements and activities, there is no need to feel unduly guilty about your lack of perfect parenting: children are great survivors!

Many of the management issues raised in this chapter will be discussed in much greater detail in Chapters 2 and 3.

References

Ambrose, N., Yairi, E. and Cox, N. (1993). Early childhood stuttering: genetic aspects. *Journal of Speech and Hearing Research* 36, 701–706.

Andrews, G. and Harris, M. (1964). *The Syndrome of Stuttering*. London: William Heinemann Medical.

Bloodstein, O. (1958). Stuttering as an anticipatory struggle reaction. In: J. Eisenson (Ed.), *Stuttering: a Symposium*. New York: Harper.

Bloodstein, O. (1970). Stuttering and normal non-fluency: a continuity hypothesis. *British Journal of Disorders of Communication* 5, 30–39.

Bloodstein, O., Alper, B. and Zisk, F. (1965). Stuttering as an outgrowth of normal disfluency. In: D. Barbara (Ed.) *New Directions in Stuttering*. Springfield: Charles C. Thomas.

Daly, D.A. (1981). Differentiation of stuttering sub-groups with Van Riper's developmental tracks: a preliminary study. *Journal of the National Student Speech–Language–Hearing Association* 9, 89–101.

Egland G.O. (1938). An analysis of repetition and prolongations in the speech of young children. Unpublished Master's thesis, State University of Iowa.

Fawcus, M. (1973). A study of the rate of absolute articulation in children and adults. Unpublished MSc thesis, University of London/Guy's Hospital Medical School.

Frewer, V. (1993). Stammering: educational implications and teacher awareness. Thesis for the Advanced Diploma in Special Needs, Gwent College of Higher Education.

Goldmann-Eisler, F. (1968) *Psycholinguistics – Experiments in Spontaneous Speech*. London: Academic Press.

Grove, T. and Walton, J. (1981). Teachers' attitudes towards stuttering. *Journal of Fluency Disorders* 6, 163–174.

Hamre, C. (1992). Stuttering Prevention 1. *Journal of Fluency Disorders* 17, 3–23.

Johnson, W. (1959). *The Onset of Stuttering*. Minneapolis: University of Minnesota Press.

Kadi-Hairifi, K. and Howell, P. (1992). Syntactic analysis of the spontaneous speech of normally fluent and stuttering children. *Journal of Fluency Disorders*, 17, 151–170.

Klein, H. and Rustin, L. (1991). Language difficulties in adolescent stutterers. *Human Communication* 1, 1.

Lass, N., Ruscello, D., Schmitt, J., Pannbacker, M., Orlando, M., Dean, K., Ruziska, J. and Bradshaw, K. (1992). Teachers' perceptions of stutterers. *Language, Speech and Hearing Services in Schools* 23, 78–81.

Lenneberg, E.H. (1967). *Biological Foundations of Language*. New York: Wiley.

Locke, J.L. (1972). Ease of articulation. *Journal of Speech and Hearing Research* 15, 194–200.

Louko, L., Edwards, M. and Conture, E. (1990). Phonological characteristics of young stutterers and their normally fluent peers: Preliminary observations. *Journal of Fluency Disorders* 15, 191–211.

McDowell, E.D. (1928). *Educational and Emotional Adjustments of Stuttering Children*. Columbia, NY: Columbia Teachers College.

Meyers, S.C. and Freeman, F.J. (1985) Mother and child speech rate as a variable in stuttering and dysfluency. *Journal of Speech and Hearing Research* 28, 346–348.

Morley, M.E. (1957) *The Development and Disorders of Speech in Childhood*. Edinburgh: Livingstone.

Nippold, M. A. and Schwarz, I.E. (1990). Reading Disorders in Stuttering Children. *Journal of Fluency Disorders* 15, 175–189.

Perkins, W.H. (1986). Discoordination of phonation with articulation and respiration. In: G.H. Shames and H. Rubin, *Stuttering Then and Now*. Columbus, OH: Charles E. Merrill.

Pindzola, R.H. (1987) . *Protocol for Differentiating the Incipient Stutterer*. Alabama: Auburn University.

Riley, G.D. and Riley, J. (1979). A component model for diagnosing and treating children who stutter. *Journal of Fluency Disorders*, 4, 279–293.

Robinson, R.J. (1987) The causes of language disorder – introduction and overview. In: *Proceedings of the First International Symposium on Specific Speech and Language Disorders in Children*. London: AFASIC.

Rommel, D., Johannsen, H.S., Schulze, H. and Hage, A. (1993). Onset, development and maintenance of childhood stuttering: preliminary results of a five year longitudinal study. Paper presented at the Third Oxford Disfluency Conference.

Starkweather, C.W. (1987). *Fluency and Stuttering*. Englewood Cliffs, NJ: Prentice-Hall.

Schonell, F. (1950). *Diagnostic and Attainment Tests*. Edinburgh: Oliver and Boyd.

St Louis, K.O., Murray, C.D. and Ashworth, M.S. (1991). Coexisting communication disorders in a random sample of school-age stutterers. *Journal of Fluency Disorders* 16, 13–23.

Van Riper, C. (1972). *The Nature of Stuttering*, 2nd edn. Englewood Cliffs, NJ: Prentice-Hall.

Wall, M.J. (1980). A comparison of syntax in young stutterers and non-stutterers. *Journal of Fluency Disorders* 5, 345–352.

Wechsler Intelligence Scale for Children (1949). New York: Psychological Co.

Weiss, A.L. and Zebrowski, P.M. (1994). The narrative productions of children who stutter: a preliminary view. *Journal of Fluency Disorders* 19, 39–63.

Williams, D.E., Melrose, B.M. and Woods, C.L. (1969). The relationship between stuttering and academic achievement in children. *Journal of Communication Disorders*, 2, 87–98.

Yairi, E. (1993). Epidemiologic and other considerations in treatment efficacy research with pre-school age children who stutter. *Journal of Fluency Disorders* 18, 197–219.

Yairi, E. and Ambrose, N. (1992). Onset of stuttering in pre-school children: selected factors. *Journal of Speech and Hearing Research* 35, 782–788.

Yairi, E. and Lewis, B. (1984). Disfluencies at the onset of stuttering. *Journal of Speech and Hearing Research* 27, 154–159.

Chapter 2
Stuttering and the Family

ROSEMARIE HAYHOW

This chapter considers a model of stuttering development that attempts to take account of the child, the family and their interactions with each other. This necessitates looking outside the traditional speech therapy literature to see how other professional groups make sense of developmental problems. Historically, speech therapy has been influenced by the medical model and so most approaches to stuttering have a greater emphasis upon the child who stutters and the details of this communication problem than is found in interactional models of developmental problems. In discussion of the model that follows, some principles that underlie therapeutic intervention are introduced along with implications for therapy.

The effectiveness of our interventions may be limited if we fail to learn from our clients. Kelly (1955), who developed a theory of personal constructs, stresses the importance of the therapist being credulous. If we allow our clients to challenge our thinking then we have to keep developing our personal and public theories about change and problems. Once we believe that we have the answer then we run the risk of making our clients fit our framework rather than developing a framework that is sufficiently flexible to allow adjustments as new ideas are presented to us via our clients and our personal study. Kelly had the courage to state that his theory was the best he could propose at the time, and that it would and should be revised in the light of new knowledge and understanding. The model discussed in this chapter is presented in the same spirit, that is, it should be expanded or refined according to the clinical evidence that individual therapists accumulate. It is offered as a preliminary framework for considering how stuttering develops within the context of the family.

Figure 2.1 presents a summary of a model of stuttering development and represents an integration of ideas.

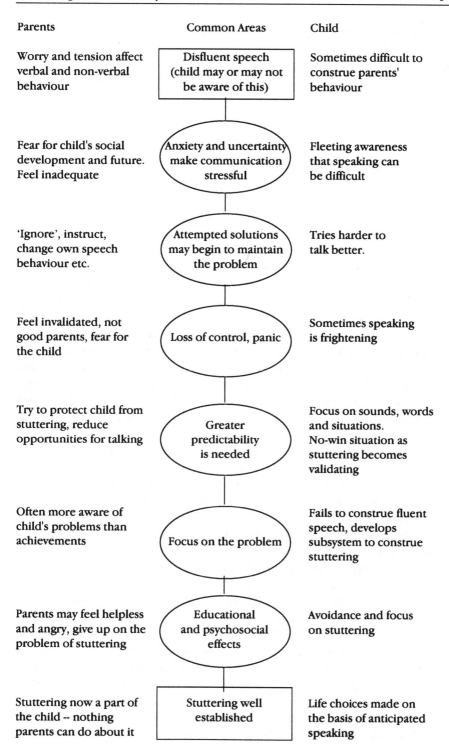

Parents	Common Areas	Child
Worry and tension affect verbal and non-verbal behaviour	Disfluent speech (child may or may not be aware of this)	Sometimes difficult to construe parents' behaviour
Fear for child's social development and future. Feel inadequate	Anxiety and uncertainty make communication stressful	Fleeting awareness that speaking can be difficult
'Ignore', instruct, change own speech behaviour etc.	Attempted solutions may begin to maintain the problem	Tries harder to talk better.
Feel invalidated, not good parents, fear for the child	Loss of control, panic	Sometimes speaking is frightening
Try to protect child from stuttering, reduce opportunities for talking	Greater predictability is needed	Focus on sounds, words and situations. No-win situation as stuttering becomes validating
Often more aware of child's problems than achievements	Focus on the problem	Fails to construe fluent speech, develops subsystem to construe stuttering
Parents may feel helpless and angry, give up on the problem of stuttering	Educational and psychosocial effects	Avoidance and focus on stuttering
Stuttering now a part of the child -- nothing parents can do about it	Stuttering well established	Life choices made on the basis of anticipated speaking

Figure 2.1. Summary of stuttering development

Elaboration of the Proposed Model of Development

The Starting Point: Awareness of Disfluent/Stuttering Speech

The starting point of this model is disfluent speech whether caused by some underlying processing difficulty, genetic predisposition, over-eagerness to talk or motor difficulty. There are good models for understanding many of the factors that can contribute to stuttering, for example Riley and Riley's Component Model (1984), Starkweather *et al.'s* Demands–Capacities model (1990) and Rommel *et al.* (1993). What we shall consider here is the way the disfluency is construed by the parents and in some instances by the child after it first occurs. Parental and clinical observation would suggest that many young children do not construe (place an interpretation upon) their disfluent speech, especially if their disfluencies arise when their attention is occupied with their emotions, desire to talk or difficulty in finding the words to complete their utterance. However, the parents whom we meet either interpret the disfluency as something negative and worrying or notice the disruptions and are not sure whether or not they signify the beginning of a bigger problem. The way that parents interpret the disfluency, or the meanings that they place upon it, are of vital importance because the way any of us understands things affects our behaviour.

Within family groups behaviours can very quickly acquire a secondary meaning or become part of an already well-established pattern. For example: the mother may interpret the disfluencies as an early sign of adult stuttering and so understandably feel very anxious, but the father may think there is nothing wrong. If this couple grew up in families where their respective mothers did the worrying about the children and the fathers distanced themselves from such concerns then they may well slip into a familiar pattern whereby the more the mother worries the more the father distances himself. This may force the mother into being more urgent in her ways of trying to get her husband to take the matter seriously. This in itself will have begun a process that enlarges rather than reduces the significance of the problem and has now become part of the difficulty that the couple have in understanding each other's points of view. It is important to realise that there is no judgement implied in the example given above; couples often behave in a complimentary manner and it is this interaction that is important.

During interviews with the parents the speech and language therapist may see this process occurring; thus so might the parents begin to understand what is happening in a new way. If the father becomes able to acknowledge the mother's concern and if, in turn, the mother can see the child's disfluencies through the father's eyes, then it is possible that both will be more respectful of each other's views and more able to offer each other appropriate support. In addition, the process of accepting that behaviour can have very different meanings for different people and may help them view the disfluency from the child's point of view. We can be pretty sure that no two and a half to three-year-old knows about stuttering and certainly would have no understanding of the long-term implications of such a way of speaking. If the parents can begin to see things in the way that their young child does then they may be able to sense both the intensity and also the transitory nature of small children's emotional reactions.

Street (1994) gives a greater priority to family members developing their understanding of each other than to the therapist's understanding of the family:

> ...it is not the counsellor's understanding that counts, it is the understanding that family members have for one another. The counsellor in providing empathic understanding to all family members offers a bridge to improved communication, a transitional step in the development of possibilities for interaction previously unavailable or unutilised in the family. (p. 31)

Extending this idea to speech and language therapy, the role of the therapist now becomes that of facilitating understanding between therapist, client, family and school staff, rather than offering advice. Providing a bridge between the different members of the family group and also between child and school has long been an aim in the author's work with adolescents who stutter.

Anxiety and Uncertainty

We have considered the child's disfluent speech and the way this is interpreted by the parents, which leads us on to explore the relationship between construing and behaviour. Children look to their parents to know what to make of things. If the message from the parents is that something is worrying then the child is likely to believe them; if the messages from the parents are conflicting then the child will be confused. If the parents do not know what to make of the problem then their behaviour may be inconsistent, making it difficult for the child to construe the parents' behaviour during disfluent speaking which in itself can lead to increased anxiety. Kelly (1955) redefined anxiety as arising when people are unable to construe the events which confront them. So the child is likely to feel anxious if he cannot construe his parents' behaviour. This cycle of behaviour and construing is shown in Figure 2.2.

When we consider the cycle shown in Figure 2.2 and then think about the interactions between different family members we begin to get a sense of the complexity of reactions and interactions that arise. It also makes it clear that what causes a particular behaviour to be a problem is not necessarily merely a matter of degree, but is much more to do with the meanings that people attach to a behaviour that determines whether

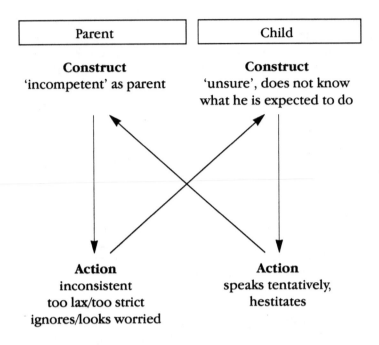

Figure. 2.2 Cycle of parent–child interaction (from Hayhow & Levy 1989)

or not it is a problem. This does not lie easily with the medical model where specific symptoms indicate a particular problem and severity is often measured by frequency, length or type of symptom. In turn, an absence of symptoms indicates successful treatment. In the stuttering literature there is a long history of attempts to differentiate between normal non-fluency and early stuttering on the basis of speech characteristics (see Chapter 1) even though most therapists recognise that this represents only a small part of the problem. Perkins (1992) differentiates between stuttering behaviour and being a stutterer and his preventive work with parents aims to stop the first leading to the second. The process of moving from being someone who *does* something to someone who *is* something (i.e. from stuttering to stutterer) is, in part, what Figure 2.1 attempts to elaborate. In therapy we may not always be able to stop the stuttering for a variety of developmental and constitutional reasons but we can aim to ensure that this does not automatically lead to becoming a stutterer. Therapy with older children and adults often addresses this problem from the other end, helping the client view him- or herself as someone who stutters rather than as a stutterer with all its negative connotations.

Attempted Solutions

It sounds like a statement of the obvious to say that for something to be a problem requiring professional intervention then it must be recognised as being a problem and, in addition, something which the person who has the problem feels unable to deal with. However, this process of problem formation is often not given sufficient thought and it may not be recognised that in most instances the people we see have tried different solutions to their child's speech problem but feel stuck and unable to deal with the problem on their own. The ideas of Watzlawick et al. (1974) on problem formation and change fit well with observations on how stuttering develops. What often happens with persisting problems is that the attempted solutions begin to maintain the problem so that the initial problem, in this case disfluency, becomes more complicated as various attempts to solve it become an intrinsic part of the problem. This process is very clearly demonstrated with established stuttering where solutions such as avoidance, increased tension and eye aversion become part of the problem.

This gradual enlargement of the problem has also been referred to as primary and secondary stuttering either in relation to specific behaviours or in relation to how handicapped the person feels by the difficulty with speaking. Often, people's attempted but unsuccessful solutions show a consistency in the way in which the problem is viewed so that these solutions are often examples of 'more of the same'. For example, a belief that stuttering is a mechanical problem, that is, a problem with saying or initiating particular sounds, will lead to a range of mechanistic type of solutions (e.g. putting more effort into production of these sounds, avoiding them or eye blinking).

The solutions in the example given above are all first-order solutions in that the problem is understood in a particular way and the solutions all follow logically from this. Second-order change involves a change in the way that the problem is viewed and so new behavioural options become possible solutions.

An example of second-order change arises when a therapist views a particular child's stuttering as a naturally occurring response to a rapid increase in linguistic skills, as a response to too much pressure to communicate at an unrealistic level or as an indication that the child has developed the mistaken belief that he needs almost constant adult attention (Dreikurs *et al.*, 1972). In the first example, possible solutions could involve informing the parents about language development and helping them differentiate between the child's experiences and their own fears. The second possibility might lead to parent counselling to help the parents be more supportive and less demanding and, in the third, the discouraged child will need to develop greater independence and so have less need for undue adult attention. All of these possible solutions have moved the focus right away from the original presenting problem, making a mechanistic solution seem inappropriate.

A therapist who wishes to grasp an appropriate second-order solution will need to explore the context in which the disfluency occurs during interviews with the parents and/or family. If we return to the first example, then this view of the child's disfluency might fit if the disfluency increased around the time of obvious development in linguistic skills and is perhaps more apparent when the child is attempting to express complex ideas, or is trying to communicate verbally when there are other pressures or demands such as tiredness, excitement or the need to speak quickly. In the second and third cases it would be important to know what happens when the child is less fluent in comparison with the more fluent episodes. The second example might be indicated when parents are very controlling in play with their child and appear rather insensitive to the child's experiences and language content. The third example might be indicated where the child receives extra attention when disfluent and where parents describe other, frequently occurring behaviours that could be construed as demands for attention. In the second two examples the therapist will need to know what happens when the child is disfluent. What does parent A do? How does parent B respond to parent A and the child? What becomes important is not just an individual parent's response to the disfluency but what that response leads to in the child and in the other family members.

These ideas have been discussed in the context of parents and child. When there are other siblings then their behaviour and the parental response to this also become important. The search for appropriate second-order solutions makes sense for therapists familiar with Fransella's (1972) work where therapy and change are viewed as a process of reconstruction; that is, the change arises initially from construing events differently, which in turn leads to changes in speaking behaviour.

Loss of Control

One of the unresolved questions about stuttering concerns why people react so negatively to it. Perkins (1992) perhaps comes close to an answer when he talks about the importance of the feelings of loss of control. Much early development is concerned with gaining control and the child who learns to control both muscles and emotions is well regarded in our society. A loss of physical and/or emotional control in a social context is looked down on or associated with psychiatric illness, learning disability or other major problems. Stuttering, by and large, is confined to social contexts and often to those interactions that the speaker and maybe parents consider in some way personally important or significant. The experience of loss of control seems to be an important landmark in the development of stuttering. Parents will often report a qualitative change in speaking behaviour as the child apparently becomes aware of difficulties in controlling his or her speech mechanisms. For some children this happens soon after the onset of disfluency, for others it happens only now and again and for some others it may never really be a problem. What can often be observed is a change from a fairly relaxed repetitive disfluency to a much more tense blocking type of stuttering accompanied by a fleeting look of fear. When parents observe their child really struggling with speaking they often feel acutely distressed and Kelly's construct of validation/invalidation seems to fit well here. Validation arises when our predictions or anticipations are proved correct by events; conversely, invalidation occurs when our predictions are proved wrong. Kelly viewed the need to make sense in order to anticipate events as a major driving force and so validation of our predictions is very important to our feelings of well-being and security. This is not the same as positive reinforcement because unpleasant events can be anticipated and hence our construing validated.

Parenting is an extremely complicated business and a trivialisation of this is not intended. However, it seems likely that most parents have a belief that if they treat their child well and if they are good enough parents then their child will develop into a reasonably happy and successful being. When a child develops a problem, and especially one that is often viewed at least in part as a psychological one (Rommel *et al.*, 1993), this brings into doubt the parents' abilities in a potentially very threatening way. The parents' notion of themselves as good enough parents is being seriously questioned. The disfluency invalidates the parents' predictions that certain behaviours on their part will produce 'normal' behaviour in their child. Invalidation is extremely unpleasant and, when it arises around events construed with very important or core constructs, the feelings of not knowing oneself can be tremendously threatening. Feeling unsure of oneself can quickly have a negative effect on family relationships so that some of the parents we see with children who are persistently disfluent are feeling extremely vulnerable. It has to be remembered that there are many factors that will affect how seriously invalidated parents feel by their child's disfluency but the more concerned they are to be good parents, the more significant the child's communicative behaviour and the more severe the child's moments of stuttering, the more likely they are to feel badly about themselves both as individuals and as parents. When one of the parents has or still does stutter themselves then feelings can become even more negative and complicated.

It is interesting how parents may change over time with regard to this problem of invalidation. For some, their repeated failed attempts to help their child speak more easily seem to lead to a shift in thinking so that gradually the child is seen as responsible for its stuttering speech. The author's clinical experience suggests that, whereas many parents of young children look for external factors to explain their child's disfluency, as time goes by they are more likely to see it as part of other negative attributes that the child has. It may be that in order for parents to be able to cope they need to separate themselves from the child's problem and that viewing stuttering as something the child does as opposed to something that happens to the child reduces their feelings of guilt and inadequacy. Changes in the parents' thinking that occur as a result of an acute problem becoming chronic are not addressed in the stuttering literature but they are undoubtedly relevant when working with the parents of stuttering children.

The Need for Predictability

It seems that the experience of loss of control can signal a new stage in the development of stuttering in that, for many, stuttering now begins to take on a much greater significance in both the child's and parents' thinking. The need to anticipate has already been discussed and the need to make some predictive sense of stuttering becomes more urgent as severity increases. Gradually the observation of when it occurs, at both a sound and situational level, leads to anticipatory behaviour. As stuttering is anticipated so its occurrence becomes validating. This places the person who stutters in a dilemma in that stuttering, whilst still hated and dreaded, becomes proof of self-knowledge and understanding, i.e. control. Similarly, if parents feel they have some ability to predict the stuttering problem they may feel less anxious and they may also begin to structure the child's experiences in such a way as to reduce the chances of stuttering. This process usually takes a long time and often it is not until puberty or adolescence that the anticipation of stuttering becomes established, and even then usually only for those who stutter severely or who for some reason are particularly sensitive to their speech difficulty.

Focus on the Problem

As time goes on there is a tendency for people to focus more and more on the problem and less and less on those times when the problem is absent or diminished (George *et al.*, 1990). This focus on the problem increases feelings of helplessness. Again there is an interesting link here with Fransella's (1972) work where she discusses how the person who stutters develops an elaborate sub-system for construing disfluent speech rather than a sort of social communication system that helps the person make sense of their own and other people's interactions. Therefore, therapy involves helping the client to construe their more fluent communications and also to become more aware of the other information available to them that will help them in the process of construing others. Just as Fransella focused therapy discussion on fluent experiences so the brief therapy school (see George *at al.*, op. cit.) aims for a shift such that the exception (i.e. fluency) no longer proves the rule but rather the exception becomes the rule.

Educational and Psychological Effects

An increasing focus on stuttering and the development of anticipatory and avoidance behaviours can lead to a constricting of a child's social and educational experiences. If we consider the pragmatic aspects first, and in particular the use of discourse skills, then there is some evidence that stuttering schoolchildren do not engage in conversations to the same extent as their non-stuttering peers. Weiss and Zebrowski (1991) obtained information from classroom teachers using a 'Discourse Skills Checklist' (Bedrosian, 1985). They found that twice as many non-stutterers as stutterers were observed to incorporate a number of the discourse features in the classroom routinely. These included, for example: 'able to make introductions'; 'able to make requests for repetitions or clarification'; 'talks about others as well as the self'; 'disagrees with others'. Only two discourse skills were found to be routinely incorporated by at least twice as many stutterers as non-stutterers: these were 'initiates a topic immediately following a topic initiation by another speaker' and 'engages in monologue when in a group'. As Weiss (1993) concludes:

> When used in conversation, both of these discourse characteristics would probably limit the participation of a speaker's co-conversationalists. (p. 221)

More studies of this type are needed if we are to appreciate the extent to which stuttering can interfere with a child's development and progress in school. This particular research supports those who work on social skills as part of therapy (e.g. Rustin, 1987) but suggests that this might be taken further to include a more thorough development of conversation skills.

If children repeatedly fail to engage in conversations in school then they will experience fewer and fewer of just those events that they need to experience if they are to develop a more sophisticated understanding of self and others. It has already been mentioned that Kelly defined anxiety as occurring when events are outside the range of a person's construct system, and so a failure to develop socially useful constructs can increase the fear and anxiety felt in difficult social situations. Jackson and Bannister's (1985) work on the development of children's construct systems suggests that in early adolescence children begin to develop more psychological constructs. Until this time they look for physical and behavioural similarities and differences between people. As they mature they begin to relate observable behaviours to underlying personality characteristics and qualities. Children who stutter severely will often judge people initially on the basis of whether they stutter or not and then ascribe characteristics to people on the basis of their fluency. It is not unusual to hear adults who stutter make statements like 'I don't understand why people who are fluent should be nervous about speaking' or 'If I hadn't a stutter I would be much more successful in life'. This is a similar phenomenon to what Van Riper (1973) refers to as the Demosothenes complex. One could argue that the person who stutters does not need to become more realistic but that rather they need to develop constructs that will help them understand themselves and others in ways that are independent of speaking abilities. When a young person has become a stutterer in the sense that their way of speaking influences their view of self and others, there are many other ways in which they may doubt themselves and we see the long-term effects in some of the adult clients who seek therapy.

This model is an attempt to look at the development of stuttering as a problem which family, friends and school contribute to, rather than a problem that resides mostly within the child. This does not lay the blame with the parents as most are doing their best but instead suggests that when stuttering persists it is a family problem and not just the child's. Perhaps in the last decade too much emphasis has been placed on the role of the parents in the development of problems within children and insufficient account taken of the effect that the child has on the parents. Parents of more than one child know that they feel differently about each child, these differences arising from the differences between the children, birth order and the relationships between the children, etc. When we take an interactional view we all have a part to play and changes in one person will have an effect on everyone else within the system. This does not discount the work that others have done on the mechanics of speaking but rather supplements that work. Whatever the underlying causes and maintaining factors of stuttering we are still left with the individuals' and families' responses to these. It is possible that when speech technique work proves to be of only short-term value that this is because the interactional aspects of stuttering have not been addressed.

Clinical Implications of the Model

The discussion so far has been rather theoretical and needs to be related to practice in order to enable the therapist to conceptualise the therapy process more clearly. There may be some conflicts between standard speech and language therapy practice and the approach derived from an integration of therapies. In order to place a particular child and family somewhere on the proposed model of development we need to gain some sense of what the problem means to them and what they are doing to cope with it. When the aim of therapy is an increase in understanding, not just for the therapist but for parents as well, then both parents and therapist need to be actively involved in the process of exploring the problem within the context of the particular family.

The First Stage of Therapy

Therapy starts as soon as the client decides he or she wishes to have therapy and all communications after that point may have an effect on outcome. The way the initial interview is conducted will set the tone for the relationship between client and therapist that is to follow, and this in turn will affect how the client views the problem, the therapy process and their role within this. The standard speech therapy case report is derived from the medical model and is concerned with an accumulation of facts that can then be interpreted by the therapist leading to a diagnosis, which in turn leads to a more or less prescribed course of therapy. The value of this approach is questionable in relation to stuttering generally, and particularly in relation to early non-fluency because one of the therapist's aims may be to assure the parents that the child's disfluency is a normal part of language development. A focus on areas of difficulty may increase awareness of shortcomings. This in turn can increase feelings of helplessness in relation to the problem. In addition, the process by which the therapist arrives at a diagnosis is often internalised in the medical model and this does little to help the parents reach a greater understanding of their particular problem with their child.

If we abandon the case history form, what are we to do? Instead of fact finding we can explore the problem through structured conversation, a skill that will need to be developed and which may not be feasible, initially, for newly qualified therapists. Although consistency throughout the interview is desirable, an insecure therapist can start with a case history and then gradually develop more conversation as he or she becomes more skilful or feels more comfortable with individual families.

The way in which the first few contacts are structured will be influenced by the therapist's preferences, the resources available and the individual family. In general, my preference is to video record the parents and pre-school child playing together in the first session, usually with one parent and then the other. This is quickly followed by a session with the parents where ample time is allowed to exchange information and discuss relevant areas, usually finishing with some clearly defined tasks or goals that lead on to the next session. When the child is older the parents and child will attend the initial interview, sometimes with other siblings. At this interview a decision is made concerning who should attend future meetings and this will depend on whether direct or indirect therapy seems appropriate. I support the view of the family therapists who welcome all those who are interested rather than those who stipulate the attendance of certain members of the family. In my experience most fathers are extremely pleased to be involved in initial therapy and it is only when therapy persists over a longish time that work pressure etc. may elect one parent as the more regular attendee. Unless we can be very flexible and offer evening and Saturday appointments the current economic and employment climate makes people nervous about missing too much time from work, so we need to be respectful of clients' constraints.

Problem Description and Definition

The initial interview may well start with some description of the parents' view of the problem and, if the child is old enough, how she and other siblings who are present view it. If the stuttering has been a problem for some time then the therapist may attempt to gain a picture of how this has changed over time. Once this historical overview has been gained, the focus should turn more onto the current problem. Street (1994) identifies two dimensions that need to be considered: the meaning dimension and the interactive dimension. The latter involves two elements:

(a) Tracking interaction around problem behaviour;
(b) Observing the interactions in the counselling room. (p. 63)

Meaning Dimension

The importance of the meaning dimension was discussed earlier and the informal elicitation of bipolar constructs provides one way of tuning into the individual differences that may exist between family members in the interpretations that they place upon behaviours and events. If the therapist listens for recurring themes then submerged poles can be verbalised by asking, in various ways, what the opposite would be (see Hayhow and Levy [1989] for fuller discussion of this approach). In this way dimensions of meaning become more apparent and differences between different individuals' construing can be explored. People may share verbal labels for one end of a construct but find the other end is different. Shared use of words, but with different meanings, is one cause of misunderstandings. During social interaction our behaviour is governed not only by our own construing but also by our construing of the others' construction processes. As problems are explored and as the therapist strives to understand each person's perspective so those present may begin to understand each other in different ways. Another feature of problem development is that individuals get stuck with their view of the problem and find it hard to shift to an alternative view. A gentle exploration of the theories that each holds regarding the problem can provide alternatives and so begin the process of change.

Interaction Dimension

Tracking interactions

The interactive dimension may be much harder for therapists to feel comfortable with than the meaning dimension. This is not because we are unaware of interaction: on the contrary, we are well trained in observing certain aspects of verbal and non-verbal communication. However, it is this training in details of communication skills that can make it difficult to take a more systemic view. Initially, it is helpful to get a broad view of the overall context into which the specific problem fits, as it is only a part of a much wider interactive pattern. Street (1994) likens interactions to streams of words which we 'punctuate' in certain ways to give particular meanings. With this analogy we can see that there is no definitive beginning or end to any particular interaction and different people may punctuate it in different ways. He goes on to say:

> ... the counsellor therefore has the task of exploring the interactive element of any reported problem and expanding the length of that interactive sequence so that the family can, in their own way, arrive at their own new punctuation. To do this they need to come to appreciate how the problem is embedded into how they interact generally. (p. 71)

In conversation with the family discussion moves from the moments of difficulty to what happens before and afterwards so that it can be seen within the context of a longer time-scale. The parents may view the child's problems with speaking as being the beginning of an interactive sequence, whereas the therapist may see the disfluency as arising in response to pressure exerted by the previous speaker. In this example the different punctuations lead to different starting points as well as different interpretations. A grandparent may see that the first speaker pressurised the child in response to a comment made by a sibling. There is always something that happened before any point that we might choose as being a starting point. What is important is not to find the true start but to consider the different meanings that arise when the starting point is moved and, in this way, to reach a new understanding.

When considering how members of a system interact we can assume that there are repeated patterns that have been set up over time. When something has been a problem for a while it is likely that family members have each settled into their own particular way of handling it. So, for example, the reluctant eater may be encouraged to eat by one parent whilst the other gets irritated by the attention that the child receives. This may lead to some snappy remark which the other parent rises to, so that parental conflict takes the attention away from the child and the food. Older children may be involved in family speaking situations that end in the stuttering child leaving the room in anger whilst everyone else is left feeling angry and guilty. These sorts of sequences can usually be readily recalled and then extended in time so that both therapist and family get a clearer view of the problem and how it fits into wider inter-active patterns. Asking what would happen if it was the father rather than the mother who was involved, or if both parents combined forces, for example, can be the beginning of finding new strategies or may reveal where previous strategies have failed.

Interactions in the Therapy Room

Observation of interactions within the therapy room will also provide information concerning usual patterns. Who represents the family, who takes control of the children, what happens when a child fails to comply? All of these types of decisions are likely to be reached and carried out in the family's usual way. The actual behaviour may not be exactly the same as would arise at home or in other situations but, generally speaking, themes and patterns will be much as usual. Parents with young disfluent children are often keen to ensure that things are not too strange and threatening for the child when they first come for therapy and so recog-nise the need to behave as they usually do to reassure the child that it is a safe situation. Interactive sequences observed in the initial sessions need to be recorded so that the therapist can build up a picture of the interactions around the problem. Requests for clarification, invitations to make additional comments and requesting comments from quieter family members can all aid the therapist's understanding but, more importantly, can help the family gain new understandings. There may also be times when the child speaks very easily and these interactions may also throw some light on the nature of the problem and suggest possible strategies for increasing fluency.

When people are stuck with a problem each may assume that the problem exists in the way that they see it, and they are not aware that each person involved has a different view. They may also assume that behaviours are motivated by the same thoughts or emotions that they experience. For example, in one family where the mother's illness resulted in very reduced mobility she felt rejected when her teenage son left the room in anger. Her son would leave the room because he could not bear stammering in front of his family and his father's requests that he finish what he was saying just made him more self-conscious about his speech. The father thought he was being encouraging but the son viewed his behaviour as punishing. The son left the room primarily to avoid the pain of not being able to say what he wanted to say and seemed genuinely unconscious of the fact that it made his mother acutely aware of her disability. The discussion of this interactive sequence and the sharing of feelings that each experienced helped this particular family to find other ways of dealing with the events that precipitated this pattern. It is my experience that the overwhelming majority of families with a child who stutters are doing the best that they can and that these repeating interactive patterns do not arise out of a desire to hurt. Very often the sharing of the different meanings that these events have for different family members leads to new options.

Variations or Fluctuations in Stuttering

Sometimes a picture emerges of a child who often stutters severely and who is gaining a considerable amount of extra attention and power as a direct result of the stuttering. Unfortunately this can happen as a result of speech and language therapists' advice to reduce all pressures and give the child extra attention. The reduction of pressures might make it difficult for the parents to clarify boundaries: this can lead to parental disagreements and family stress as the child becomes almost too power-ful within the family. The parents are so relieved when the child is more fluent and so depressed and disheartened when the child is stuttering that they will treat the child very differently from other children in their attempts to reduce stuttering. Sometimes there are other problems, maybe with eating or sleeping, which increases the parents' anxiety and makes them even more fearful of clarifying boundaries for the child. It is not that the young child is doing all this intentionally but rather that he has drawn the wrong conclusions from the behaviour of the adults around him. It is as if he feels at a loss if he is not the centre of attention.

One couple who were describing a typical interaction that involved their middle child started to be able to draw some boundaries as a result of being asked to repeat an utterance. The mother said, 'she won't even let me have a cup of coffee', she being the three-year-old disfluent child. The therapist put on a pretence of not hearing, though the non-verbal cues made it clear to the mother that she had heard and that the repeti-tion was for the mother's sake. When the mother said it again both she and her husband laughed with relief at their shared realisation that the child did not need to dictate her mother's coffee-drinking habits and that it could not in any way be a benefit to the child to be making such decisions. The mother left determined to drink a cup of coffee when she wanted to the following morning. The next week it transpired that the mother had kept her promise to herself; she had the resources to take such a decision and both parents had begun to find ways of dealing more effectively with the children. Over the next few sessions they began to explore ways of taking better care of each other as well as responding to the different needs of their children. The child's fluency, eating and sleeping all began to improve. The change in the mother after four sessions was striking in that she was much more relaxed, more assertive and seemed much happier. She felt she was taking the demands of the children more in her stride and she had begun to lower some of the high expectations she had for herself. This particular child had received a great deal of attention because of her difficult behaviour, allergies etc. and this had also made it difficult for the parents to see her as a normal, strong and very determined little girl. The child attended only the initial speech therapy session when she spoke fluently, with precocious language skills, well-structured and imaginative play and was generally a delight to meet. When a child, who can be very difficult with his or her parents, can handle a potentially threatening situation with such ease it does suggest that the child is an expert at handling adults. Such children can easily be seen as manipulative or over-demanding but such judgements may lead the therapist to take sides, something that needs to be avoided if the aim is to view the family as a system. No one person can be held responsible for the problems that arise within the system: they are a function of the system and as such everybody has a part to play.

Other Assessments and Information

When the child's pattern of disfluency is more consistent with an underlying language problem, further assessment may be required. However, this begs the question of whether a language difficulty would ever in itself account for stuttering. Interestingly, clinical evidence suggests that very few children with language difficulty have a persisting problem with stuttering and that problems such as dyspraxia where disfluency is apparent do not usually require the disfluency to be addressed as an issue separate from the intelligibility problems. Studies that have looked at the role of language in stuttering have usually found oral motor problems to be more apparent, though unfortunately some of these studies do not differentiate between phonological and motor problems (e.g.. Riley and Riley, 1984; Rommel *et al.,* 1993). Whatever the evidence for and against a language element in stuttering we are still left with the important issue of how the child and family deal with the disfluency. Put another way, the underlying causal factors may be less important in determining outcome than the degree of understanding and support that the child experiences in his or her environment. Where a child has a speech or language problem that is obvious to the highly trained eyes and ears of the therapist then this must be addressed, as it would be unrealistic to expect the child to become more fluent when the process of transferring ideas into words is problematic. However, when the underlying difficulty is subtle and when very detailed assessment is required to unearth it then one can argue that the first line of action must be to ensure that the child's environment is maximally supportive and that the pressures or rewards that could maintain a stuttering problem are removed. This would not only provide the best possible context for the development of fluency but also provide a good language environment. If the disfluency persists when all the interactional factors have been addressed then perhaps this is the time for deeper investigation.

The tension that exists between the medical and interactional/family models is not necessarily a bad thing. We do not have to reject completely the old in favour of the new but rather should be guided by the hypotheses that we formulate as our understanding of a particular client increases. It is possible to obtain case history-type information without working through the standard format. The drawing of a family tree (Barker, 1986) invites discussion about different family members and families will often volunteer information that they consider important in relation to particular family members. Consideration of the client's stage in the family life cycle (Dare, 1979) provides a good picture of stresses and supports as well as providing indicators of possible adjustment problems. Discussion of the parents' beliefs concerning the cause and nature of the problem will usually lead to descriptions of any relevant traumatic events that the child and/or family have experienced.

Recorded observation of the child and parents playing together can provide information on interactions and also provide data for speech and language analysis. Analysis of the nature and severity of the disfluency, when it arises, what happens immediately before and after, as well as more general information concerning the focus of the play session and the relevance of the language to the child's activity can all be completed at a later stage if deemed necessary.

There are advantages in allowing the client some responsibility in leading the direction of the early sessions, for example:

- The clients' version of their story is respected; they are in charge of what they disclose.
- When the aim is increased understanding the therapist will ask questions for clarification, and the parents may begin to see things differently without areas being probed that the parents would not volunteer to discuss.
- The process of getting to know and understand need not highlight problems and weaknesses within the family relationships.
- Problems will emerge but they need not be excessively focused on in the initial interview. If we are really striving for an equal relationship with the parents we work with, then they must feel some control over the content of the session.
- If the ultimate aim of therapy is autonomy then sharing responsibility from the outset addresses issues of power in the therapeutic relationship.
- One aim of therapy is to find better ways of handling the problem and this can be done only by sharing the resources that the therapist and family have to offer. By encouraging clients to take an active role from the beginning we can gain an understanding of the resources they have by seeing some of these in action in the clinic room. For exam-

ple, how they discuss the problem together, how they reach shared understanding and how they handle disagreement.

Working towards Change

When the family is viewed as a system there is no 'correct' or 'right' way for parents to behave with their children. Consideration of the interactions that occur around instances of disfluent speech may lead the parents to decide to alter their responses but this will be done on the basis of a particular system and not because the therapist has some notion of an ideal communication environment. The parents can then evaluate for themselves whether or not the altered behaviour was helpful to the child and, if not, they can experiment with something else. We have already discussed how one feature of problem development is getting stuck with a particular set of responses, behaviours or way of viewing things. Feeling free to begin some careful experimentation can be the start of regaining some predictive control. Care should be taken not to try too many different responses in too short a space of time because inconsistent parental responses could increase a child's anxiety. However, parental discussion and reflection on more fluent speaking may help them develop responses that facilitate fluency in their own child.

We do not have research evidence to support the accepted wisdom of encouraging parents to refrain from any direct reference to the child's speaking problem or that they should avoid giving any advice to the child concerning alterations in manner of speaking. There is plenty of clinical evidence to be found in the form of adults' recollections that pretending to ignore stuttering is unhelpful. There are many adults who stutter who never discussed their speech with their parents and who find trying to break the conspiracy of silence extremely difficult. However, there are parents who report positive results when they suggest that their child slows down or starts again and this raises questions about whether it is the particular type of stuttering problem that renders these types of suggestion helpful or whether it is the matching of the parents' particular suggestion with the child's problem at that particular moment that is important.

It seems unreasonable to stop parents from trying to help a child who may be quite obviously struggling and aware of that struggle. If parents can be encouraged to try to see the speaking situation from the child's point of view they may be able to offer appropriate help. For example, if the child is obviously upset about something that has happened then some comment on the child's speech would diminish the child's emotional experience which could increase frustration. On the other hand, a parental comment that reflects the child's intensity of feelings may help reduce this intensity and so help the child say what is necessary. Conversely, when a child is struggling to express an abstract idea in complex language, then they may be helped either by indicating that there is no hurry or by questions that enable the child to structure his or her ideas. Another possibility is that the parents realise that the increased disfluency is a result of tiredness and over-excitement, and so a bath and an early night with familiar bedtime stories may be the best remedy. This type of approach encourages parents to tune in more carefully to their child's needs and to then respond creatively or intuitively rather than to try and remember expert advice on what to do.

When discussing this idea with parents an analogy can be used to help them conceptualise the sort of intervention that might be helpful. It is important that if parents are to try to help their child they must use their own language so that it feels and sounds natural to them all. One such analogy could be with running and falling. When a child falls and is genuinely hurt most parents go quickly to the child and perform the necessary checking and comforting rituals. If the child falls and makes a lot of noise but the parents feel sure that he is not hurt they will not over-react but encourage more independence from the child. Alternatively the parents may notice that it is getting late and that the child keeps tripping up, and realise they must hurry home to food, bath and bed. These different responses arise automatically from the parents' interpretations of the child's verbal and non-verbal behaviours. It seems likely that parents are free to respond in these different ways because they have no fear of their child growing into a chronic, adult knee-grazer. They are free to respond to the child in the present without undue regard for the effect that today's response will have on the child's future as an adult. Encouraging parents to tune into their child's thinking and experiences is one way in which they can be helped to remain in the present while their child speaks disfluently.

Encouraging this type of tuning in can also help parents become more sensitive to their child's communication and thought processes. For those parents who have no knowledge of child development, and no recent experience of young children, it can be very difficult for them to differentiate between their own thinking and the sort of thought processes that arise in young children. In particular they may have difficulty in appreciating how concrete children are in their thought processes. This misunderstanding is demonstrated when parents ask children about what they did at playgroup or with another adult/child without providing any cues or associations to make the task less abstract.

Finding ways to help parents tune in more finely to their children is an example of promoting second-order change. Parents are not given specific behavioural directives, such as to speak more slowly, simplify their language or ask fewer questions. We are easily made to feel more inadequate when it is suggested that we change a behaviour which is not readily, consciously changed. It is interesting that Procter *et al.* (1987)

discuss how first-order change is often difficult to achieve, requiring hard work and discipline, whereas second-order change can arise with little conscious effort. So parents can be given tasks that will encourage them to get on the same wavelength as their child in the expectation that changes in behaviour will follow automatically. The tasks might be observational, they might involve talking to another parent or perhaps looking at children's books in the library and trying to anticipate which their child will select and enjoy. Whenever possible, second-order change is preferable in that it avoids repeating a pattern of failure and then setting up yet more solutions that might maintain the problem. It is also important to try to avoid the trap of more of the same that has already failed. It is not just that one is always looking for an easy way out but rather that one is attempting to channel energies into understanding and creativity rather than setting up patterns that are doomed to failure.

This chapter has attempted to elaborate a picture of how stuttering develops within a family context and to show how an integration of ideas from different theoretical backgrounds influences both therapy structure and content. A consideration of how stuttering is developing within the family, how it is affecting individual members and how it affects their interactions gives a different structure to initial exploration of the problem from the conventional type of assessment. Therapy can aim to address not just the observable features of the problem but also the psychological and interactional dimensions in which the problem is also developing. It is hoped that this chapter gives a flavour of therapy: a more detailed account of what therapy could entail at the different levels or stages of development would take much longer. In particular, when considering the older child it is not just the family system that is relevant but also the school and friendship systems as well as the child's psychological development. Kelly (1955) refers to man as the scientist; the child's developing role as scientist can be severely limited if too many of life's experiments focus upon speech fluency at the expense of other more socially useful constructions. Thus this is by no means a complete picture and much more work needs to be done if we are really to understand how stuttering develops and is maintained within the family and at school. As our understanding of this process increases we may become more successful in our interventions.

References

Barker, P. (1986). *Basic Family Therapy*. London: Collins.

Bedrosian, J. (1985). An approach to developing conversational competence. In: D. Ripich and F. Spinelli (Eds), *School Discourse Problems*. San Diego: College Hill Press.

Dare, C. (1979). Psychoanalysis and systems in family therapy. *Journal of Family Therapy* 1, 137–151.

Dreikurs, R. and Soltz, V. (1972). *Happy Children: A Challenge to Parents*. London: Fontana.

Fransella, F. (1972). *Personal Change and Reconstruction*. London: Academic Press.

George, E., Iveson, C. & Ratner, H. (1990). *Problem to Solution: Brief Therapy with Individuals and Families*. London: Brief Therapy Press.

Hayhow, R. and Levy, C. (1989). *Working with Stuttering: A Personal Construct Therapy Approach*. Bicester, Oxon: Winslow Press.

Jackson, S. and Bannister, D. (1985). The development of self-construing in children. Unpublished paper.

Kelly, G. (1955). *The Psychology of Personal Constructs*, Vols 1 and 2. New York: Norton.

Perkins, W. (1992). *Stuttering Prevented*. London: Whurr Publishers.

Peters, T. and Guitar, B. (1991). *Stuttering: An Integrated Approach*. Baltimore: Williams & Wilkins.

Procter, H. and Walker, G. (1987). Brief therapy. In: E. Street (Ed.), *Family Therapy in Britain*. New York: Harper & Row.

Riley, G. and Riley, J. (1984). A component model for treating stuttering in children. In: M. Peins (Ed.), *Contemporary Approaches in Stuttering Therapy*, (pp.123–171). Boston, MA: Little, Brown.

Rommel, D., Johannsen, H., Schulze, H. and Hage, A. (1993). Onset, development and maintenance of childhood stuttering: A five year longitudinal study – preliminary results. Paper presented at the Third Oxford Disfluency Conference.

Rustin, L. (1987). *Assessment and Therapy Programme for Disfluent Children*. Windsor: NFER Nelson

Starkweather, W., Gottwald, S. and Halfond, M. (1990). *Stuttering Prevention: a Clinical Method*. Englewood Cliffs, NJ: Prentice-Hall.

Street, E. (1994). *Counselling for Family Problems*. London: Sage.

Van Riper, C. (1973). *The Treatment of Stuttering*. Englewood Cliffs, NJ: Prentice-Hall.

Watzlawick, P., Weakland, J. and Fisch, R. (1974). *Change: Principles of Problem Formation and Problem Resolution*. New York: Norton.

Weiss, A. and Zebrowski, P. (1991). *A comparison of classroom discourse competencies of stuttering and nonstuttering students*. Paper presented to annual convention of the American Speech–Language–Hearing Association, Atlanta.

Weiss, A. (1993). *The pragmatic context of children's disfluency*. Seminars in Speech and Language 14(3).

Chapter 3
Working with Young Children

ROSEMARIE HAYHOW

In this chapter we consider approaches to therapy with children who continue to stutter after environmental and interactional factors have been addressed. The aim of this chapter is to explore some of the implications of different therapies and to raise questions rather than support or reject particular approaches. It is assumed that we still do not know enough about stuttering to be able to dictate the form that therapy should take and that because it is a complex and variable problem different children will respond positively to different approaches. Mater (1993), in her discussion of the neural basis of language, suggests that:

> Since so many systems need to be co-ordinated, over time and in the context of developmental, genetic, hormonal, and environmental factors, stuttering might emerge from a variety of sources or mechanisms, consistent with the heterogeneity that is seen in the research on this population. In addition, stuttering is not only developed in, but appears to be maintained by social context and emotional factors. (p. 21)

If we agree with this view and we then add to these variables other therapist and therapy variables it is clear that we are not in a position to be dogmatic. I think I have given up trying to know all that is known about stuttering but I have not given up trying to understand how stuttering develops and how this process can be halted and redirected. So I hope the reader will question what is written and that this will stimulate further thinking and development.

Current Approaches with Young Stuttering Children

Two methods will be described that have a different approach towards the child's speech but take a similar and currently accepted view of the parents' role in the maintenance of stuttering. The first method aims to modify the child's stuttering to a simpler form whereas the second trains the child to speak fluently. There will be continued debate concerning the relative merits of the 'stutter more fluently' vs 'speak more fluently' (Gregory, 1979) approaches and as yet we have no clear guidelines that help in the choice of one approach over another for a particular child. However, if the child speaks slowly and is distressed by his stuttering then modification of the actual stuttering would seem more appropriate than an approach which could be seen to be avoiding the need to cope with the stuttering. One possible hypothesis for a child like this is that he is over-sensitive to his fluency failure and perhaps also generally lacking in confidence. Experiencing a loss of control while speaking would be particularly painful for a child like this and so work on desensitisation, learning how to regain control over speaking and plenty of varied and positive speaking experiences might help. Work with the parents might involve finding ways of increasing the child's confidence and this may need to be done, in the first instance, by helping the parents to feel more confident.

Alternatively a child may speak rapidly, get very excited over relatively small disruptions, events etc. and seem largely unaware of stuttering: in this case fluency training may be the preferred approach. A possible hypothesis is that a child like this often suffers from an overloading of the system and therapy needs to help him find ways of reducing the linguistic load by, for example, slowing adult speech rate, encouraging the child to hold back by working on turn taking and by working with the parents to increase the child's tolerance for disruption. This might involve a more regular routine at home, more sleep for the child and a playing down of exciting events.

Of course, many children will fall between these extremes and an integrated approach of the sort described by Peters and Guitar (1991) may be appropriate. Alternatively, the therapist may bide her time by working first with the parents to develop an encouraging language environment where difficulties can be discussed in an open and relaxed manner, and only when this fails to achieve changes in fluency work directly with the child. By this time, both therapist and parents may be able to select the best approach for the child based on the knowledge gained during the time spent working with the parents. Two approaches that give a good indication of the sort of direct work that is being done with young children and their parents will now be described. This leads on to discussion of some of the issues and questions raised by these two programmes.

Demands Capacities Model (DCM)

Capacities

In the DCM model approach (Starkweather *et al.*, 1990) assessment aims to identify any weaknesses in the child's capacity for fluency and any demands for fluency that are unrealistic or unattainable for the particular child. The capacities for fluency fall into four main areas: motor speech control; language formulation; social-emotional maturity; and cognitive skill.

Motor speech control: The possibility of the stuttering child having problems in the area of speech motor skill was presented by Riley and Riley (1984) in their component model when they found that 87% of their sample had 'oral motor disorders'. More recently, the work of Rommel *et al.* (1993) suggests that 60% of children have some degree of motor problems. Starkweather *et al.* particularly mention the child's ability to coordinate movements at speed affecting the child's rate of syllable production.

Language formulation: This area is subdivided into word-finding, the formulation of grammatical sentences and knowledge of conversational rules. Minor problems with these aspects of language production are common in young children during periods of rapid linguistic development and are usually associated with normal disfluencies. The authors argue that, for a child already under pressure, difficulties in these areas could lead to excessive disfluency.

Social-emotional maturity: Development in this area may influence the child's ability to deal with factors such as excitement, competition to speak and relationships with peers as well as their willingness to separate from their carers whilst at school and their independence, amongst other things.

Cognitive skill: The authors are interested in metalinguistic skills but with particular reference to girls' apparent ability to recover from stuttering at an earlier age, and presumably sooner after onset, than boys. They cite the work of Yairi (1982) who found a sex ratio among very young stutterers of 1:1 and of Seider *et al.* (1983) who suggest a sex-linked, genetic predisposition to recover from stuttering. Their clinical experience of teaching metalinguistic skills to young children to help them cope with stuttering also supports the idea that girls acquire these earlier and more easily than boys.

Demands

Time pressure: The term 'time pressure' is used to cover a wide range of communicative pressures, not only the obvious ones like rapid rate of adult speech, interruptions, finishing child's sentence, rushed household environment and so on. They also include parental speech characterised by adult vocabulary and complex syntax and go on to suggest that such language places two kinds of demands on the child. These are:

> (1) the longer word takes more time to find and the more complex sentence more time to formulate, and (2) the longer items are more difficult to plan and execute. (Starkweather *et al.*, 1990, p. 17)

There are pragmatic variables that might influence the amount of choice or spontaneity that the child experiences. When a lot of questions are asked the child is frequently in the position of having to speak and to do so within a short period of time. Questions also demand that the respondent thinks about whatever is in the mind of the questioner which may require additional thinking time when compared with the formulation of spontaneous utterances. However, it is noted that questions can be phrased so that the respondent need say very little or is free to elaborate if they wish. For example, the child is freer with a 'did you enjoy...?' question than with a 'tell me what you did' directive.

Excitement: This emotion is well recognised as a fluency disrupter for many children and it is suggested that two or three factors may combine to influence the child's speech production. First, when the child is excited, speech tends to be more rapid; second, the emotional experience distracts from the linguistic task and, third, excitement may interfere with motor planning and coordination.

Interruptions: Interrupting the child has been mentioned but the child may also wish or need to interrupt. It is usual for some sort of disfluency to fill the period of overlap which must then be followed by a rapid completion of the utterance once the other speaker has stopped.

Uncertainty: This may result from important changes in the child's life at home or outside, in school or day care, and can have a negative effect on a child who is passing through a vulnerable phase or is at risk for disfluency.

Avoidance: A need to avoid stuttering can arise when a child gets negative messages about his speaking. Because many young children do not have the verbal skills to change words they may deal with this pressure by avoiding speaking or by trying harder to speak more fluently, quickly leading to increased tension and physical pressure.

During assessment and then in therapy the clinician may modify his or her communication style to facilitate fluency. Initially this enables the therapist to observe the effect that specific changes in adult speech have upon the particular child and then to model those that facilitate fluency to the parents. These fluency enhancers include:

1. Slow, stretched speech, with normal intonation.
2. Simple, short sentences.
3. Many silent periods.
4. Elimination of questions, interruptions and demands for verbal performance.
5. Use of slowed conversation, turn-taking style.
6. Use of self-talk and parallel play.
7. Following the child's lead in play.
8. Producing normal non-fluencies during conversation.(Starkweather *et al.*, 1990, p. 46)

Direct work with the child starts with open discussion of stuttering at a level appropriate to the child's age and assumed level of awareness.

Therapy then aims to work backwards from the child's stage of stuttering to the relaxed repetitions of normal disfluency. This is done primarily by modelling an easy stuttering pattern which the child is encouraged to use once she has learnt to identify his moments of stuttering. The therapist's open attitude towards stuttering aims to make it easier for the parents to talk to their child about speaking difficulties and also desensitises both parents and child to fluency failure.

In most cases, parental speaking and communication with their children is worked on in parent groups and information and advice is given concerning relevant areas of child development. The parent sessions are organised using Egan's (1986) three-stage process: identifying problems, brainstorming possible solutions and choosing a solution. The therapist takes an active listening role, asks open questions and reflects feelings. Areas or issues that are commonly identified as problematic are discussed. Some examples are given below:

1. Excessive demands are reduced by substituting modelling and providing a commentary which the parents observe when the therapist works with the child. It seems likely that other aspects of the parent sessions may influence attitudes, which in turn might help them tune in to their child more effectively.

2. Lack of confidence in the child is tackled by advising parents to ensure a special, uninterrupted talking time so that the child receives the full attention of one parent at least once a day. Fifteen minutes is the recommended time and any activity that can be enjoyed together is suitable.

3. The reduction of interruptions is considered important and so conversational rules that will facilitate turn taking are discussed with the parents and implemented by them at home. This may be as simple as stating that interrupting is rude, and both parents and children are discouraged from doing it. In larger families, where competition to speak is more pressing, some more formalised turn-taking rules may need to be used until the child is more fluent.

4. Negative parental responses to disfluency are gradually replaced by more positive ways of dealing with the underlying anxiety. Many parents are placed in a bind when instructed to ignore a child's disfluency. They may manage to suppress any verbal comments about the child's speech but they may not be able to suppress non-verbal messages, which are likely to arise too quickly and spontaneously for the parent to inhibit. Thus the child receives mixed messages. To try to deal with this problem parents are trained to recognise negative, non-verbal behaviours and then gradually to start reflecting back to the child some of the emotions and difficulties connected with speaking. This can be done at times when the child is obviously aware and bothered by his speech. Being able to respond in an open and

supportive manner helps the parents reduce their negative non-verbal responses and also allows the child to comment on speaking difficulties.

This approach has been described in some detail because the DCM has been influential in thinking and therapy for young stuttering children and combines many aspects of accepted current knowledge about stuttering. The model is relatively easy to conceptualise, so therapists can devise their own methods for assessing and working on these different areas. There are points to discuss concerning this approach, which will be considered along with points arising from the approach of Meyers and Woodford.

The Fluency Development System (TFDS) for Young Children (ages 2–9 years)

The TFDS programme (Meyers and Woodford 1992) was developed from the diagnostic approach outlined by Gregory and Hill (1980). Video recordings of each parent playing with the child are used to obtain a detailed description of the child's communication skills, fluency failures, and the parents' interaction styles with the child. The child's communication skills are assessed to determine level of development and to identify any particular problems. In many ways, this approach is similar to that taken in DCM outlined above. Parent–child interaction is analysed for interruptions, speaking rate, positive and negative utterances, questions, comments and imperatives. Turn taking is also analysed, first at the level of initiation and termination and then in terms of the time spent interacting and the number of turns.

Children diagnosed as *normally disfluent* would not be taken on for fluency training but the parents would receive support, and guidance on modifications that they can make to the child's communication environment. The parents of the stuttering child are worked with in similar ways but over a longer period of time and the child is taken on for therapy. Therapy with children is based on cognitive-behavioural principles and they learn three basic rules: use slow speech to talk more efficiently; practise smooth speech to talk more easily; and take turns to avoid interrupting and to give the speaker ample time to communicate a message. The programme provides story books, equipment and ideas for activities to teach and elaborate the slow/fast, smooth/bumpy and turn-taking concepts. This is done in ways very similar to the concept teaching in Metaphon Therapy (Howell and Dean, 1991) for children with phonological problems and therapists familiar with this approach should find it relatively easy to develop their own ideas and equipment to teach the fluency enhancing/reducing concepts.

The first stage of therapy resembles Ryan's (1974) Gradual Increase in Length and Complexity (GILCU) programme with the inclusion of the three fluency concepts. Slow/fast is taught at the 1–2 word level, smooth/bumpy at the 2–4 word level and turn taking with the 5-word–conversation level. Once the child is comfortable with speaking smoothly and slowly and in taking turns with the slow, smooth-speaking therapist then the idea of pressure is introduced and the child is gradually toughened up for the pressures of speaking outside. The child is taught ways of dealing with Mr Pressure. Once the child is sufficiently practised in the skills identified so far then the parents are introduced into the therapy setting.

Prior to joining the session the parents and clinician practise fluency-enhancing techniques (e.g. slowing down, pausing before taking a turn, commenting not questioning or whatever else was identified as being a contributory behaviour). Parents then plan a five-minute play session with the child which the therapist monitors and provides very specific feedback on. The clinician reinforces the parent when the following are noted:

1. (Parent) provides reinforcement when the child is slow and/or smooth;
2. uses a slow and/or smooth speech model; and
3. does not criticise, interrupt, or ask open-ended questions. (Meyers and Woodford, 1992, p. 79)

Therapy to this stage can take as long as eight months of weekly sessions and these are gradually reduced if the child maintains fluency. The programme is very detailed and appears to have been designed to be followed easily by generic speech and language therapists and not just by those with specialist knowledge and skills.

Topics are listed for 'behaviouristic counselling' where the aim is to provide information in a straightforward, unemotional way. 'Parents are encouraged to share because the counselor is laying the foundation for more humanistic conversations later in the course of counseling' (Meyers and Woodford, 1992, p.125). Twelve topics are suggested including language and general development, stuttering, the therapy techniques, discipline and helping the child express feelings.

The time taken to work through the programme and the detailed focus upon speaking do raise questions concerning its appropriateness for very young children or for those who are older but not concerned by their stuttering. The child's suitability for the programme seems to be determined by the type and extent of disfluency exhibited in clinic. The relatively late stage (i.e. after 6–7 months) at which the parents are taught fluency-enhancing techniques rules out the possibility of achieving fluency by environmental manipulation rather than by direct focus on the child. It is not clear in the manual at which stage the parents attend the parent counselling group. If this happens before the direct therapy then this would address the comment above. However, if it happens at the same time then it is impossible to evaluate whether it is the parent counselling, the direct work with the child or a bit of both that leads to the changes in the child's speech. This is an important point, as weekly therapy over eight months could involve a child missing half a day a week of school for the equivalent of an academic year, which requires a considerable commitment from both parents and child.

In this behavioural programme the therapist is provided with enough detail and materials to run the treatment in the prescribed manner and maintain firm control on both the child and parents. Although this control is relaxed to some extent during the counselling sessions there is still a very definite agenda that the therapist works through. It would appear that the therapist is very much the expert and that therapy is programme rather than client led. The manual is a very useful resource and the work is well referenced so that at times it reads as much like a textbook as a therapy programme.

Some Considerations when Selecting Therapeutic Approach

Theoretical Orientation

There may be confusion when a therapist who has previously been working with parents at the level of the family system then begins to work directly with the child. Two very different models are being used, one that says the problem is part of the family interaction patterns and the other that the problem resides within the child. One way of looking at this dilemma is to focus again on the family as an interactive and reactive system, thus stressing that the way parents behave is as much a function of the child as it is of the parents. When aspects of a child's behaviour are upsetting or cause problems this will inevitably affect the behaviour of the parents and other siblings. How they behave will be influenced not only by the specific behaviour but also by the interpretations that are placed on the behaviour. From this line of argument it could follow that if there are factors within the child that are leading to the problem behaviour then, when possible, these need to be addressed so that the family interactions become more satisfying for all members.

The Parent–Therapist Relationship

The role of the parents in therapy needs to be clarified if both parents and therapist are to know what is expected of them. There are at least three possibilities, which have been termed the expert, transplant and consumer models (Cunningham and Davis, 1985). In the first and probably currently least favoured model, the therapist as expert works with the child and the parents are only minimally involved. In the transplant model the parents are taught certain skills by the therapist which they incorporate into their general communicative behaviour or use during special speaking sessions. The consumer model uses the skills, knowledge and understanding of both therapist and parents to find the best ways of handling the current problem.

In the literature on young children the transplant model is probably the most commonly used, with parents being taught fluency-enhancing speaking styles in line with the direct work being done with the child. When the transplant model is used the therapist will decide which parental behaviours are to be modified and then teach the parent or draw the parents' attention to these behaviours. An example of this approach is found in the Meyers and Woodford (1992) programme, described above. Utterances are classified according to whether they are (1) interruptions; (2) positive or negative interactions; (3) questions; (4) comments; (5) imperatives. The percentage of parental utterances that are accounted for by each of the above categories is then computed. Interestingly it is only in the analysis of interruptions that the child's and conversational partner's disfluency is recorded. This approach highlights some of the problems with the transplant model in that the knowledge and expertise of the therapist is what governs the assessments and their interpretations. In this particular instance some balance in the different types of interactions is aimed for and yet the effects of these interactions on the child's fluency are not assessed. In the programme manual, details and a summary of a case are provided and comments are made about the child's response to questioning by the father. However, it could be argued that there is insufficient breakdown of the data to support the recommendation that the father should reduce the number of questions asked. If the therapist were to work according to the consumer model, she would need to share her knowledge about the sort of speech and conversation styles that facilitate fluency contrasted with those that reduce fluency. The next step would be to look at interaction data obtained from video recordings to see how the therapist's knowledge fitted with the particular child and parents. This would also need to be compared with the parents' perceptions of what influences the child.

Botterill *et al.* (1991) describe an approach that helps parents to identify their interaction styles and then modify these as seems appropriate. This alone has led to encouraging results with many of the preschool children with whom they worked. Although there are fewer data on how parental speech is affected by their child's stuttering it may be that some of the behaviours found in parents of children with language delay are relevant and that a similar approach can be taken with the parents of disfluent or language-delayed children.

The adoption of the expert model has led to problems when evaluating the effectiveness of therapy. It is generally agreed that speech in the therapy context is likely to be more fluent than in the person's everyday life, especially when therapy involves direct work on speech. However, when the therapists are the experts then they are the ones who must evaluate effectiveness. In the past this has led to discussions of some rather complicated ways of collecting speech data without the knowledge and consent of the speaker (e.g. Ingham, 1985) this being the logical extension of therapist as expert. When it is child speech data that are being collected the picture is even more confused as many experience episodic stuttering and also many are more fluent in clinic than at home, where there may be real competition to speak, excitement, frustration and so on. In addition, if parental anxiety is an element in the maintaining factors then the fact that they are with the therapist may have an effect on the child's speech. It is possible that for the first time ever the parents want the child to stutter in order to demonstrate the severity of the problem. Paradoxically this may help the child to speak fluently because the parents will not be doing anything to try to stop the stuttering. They are also in a position where they can briefly suspend their anxiety because they are with someone whom they hope will have an answer to their problems. How strong an influence these factors will have on the child's speech will depend upon the extent to which the parents' attempted solutions are maintaining the problem and, conversely, the extent to which the child's disfluency is caused and maintained by factors within the child. Evaluation of therapy becomes a little easier when the client or parents are viewed as partners in the therapeutic venture. Their view and experiences must be taken into account when assessing progress and, although this may not make objective evaluation for research or audit purposes any more straightforward, at least for clinical purposes we can justify the use of subjective data from various sources.

There are other reasons for taking the consumer or partnership model seriously, not least to guard against the over-generalisations that can occur when a particular belief takes on the status of truth because of its frequent citation in the literature. A current case in point is that of the significance of questions directed at the child. In Chapter 1, Fawcus takes a historical view of early stuttering and the possible role of excessive parental demands. It seems reasonable that parents who are over-demanding, or who generally wish to maintain control of the conversation rather than follow the child's lead, are likely to be difficult conversation partners for the young child. However, we know that not all questions require the same sort of answers and that some may make speaking easier for the child. For example, forced alternatives narrow the child's choices and also allow her to copy the desired response. To class 'would you like juice or milk?' as being in the same category as 'why did you hit your baby brother?' ignores both emotional and linguistic factors. The idea that questions can be graded according to the level of demand that they make of the respondent was used as the basis for the Stocker Probe Technique (Stocker, 1980) and although this assessment has been criticised for not taking enough account of length of response as well as other demands, it nevertheless makes us aware of how varied questions can be and the variety of possible responses. A therapist who believes the parents to be experts on their own child will listen to what they have to say concerning factors that influence fluency. Through discussion and joint viewing of video data, for example, they will discover the specific pragmatic influences on fluency. In this way, the consumer model encourages professionals to always evaluate their academic and practical knowledge in the light of particular clients rather than make the clients fit their knowledge or preferred therapy programme. This applies whatever the theoretical background of the therapist, and those using client-centred approaches are not immune from this particular abuse of client confidence.

The model of professional/client relationship that the therapist works with has implications for all aspects of therapy and consistency in approach at different stages of therapy can help the therapist structure his or her work and help clarify for the parents the role they have in relation to the child's problem and therapy.

The Modification of Parental Communication Behaviour

In the last 15 years parents have been increasingly involved in therapy and there is a general consensus that this has had a positive effect on their children's speech. However, there has been very little research that has attempted to either sort out what it is that has been helpful or what effects therapist advice has on parental behaviour. The brief therapy school are interested to know 'what is the difference that makes a difference?' (Bateson, 1972) as by knowing this it becomes possible to reduce therapy time without inevitably compromising outcome. Shorter spells of therapy can also reduce the risk of setting up dependent relationships. When therapy involves work with parents and children, both together and separately, there are so many things going on at the same time that it can be very difficult to sort out what has had the therapeutic effect. Some research that attempts to unravel some of these problems will be considered.

Reducing Parental Rate of Speech

We cannot always predict how attempts to modify one behaviour may affect other related behaviours. An interesting study by Ratner (1993) found that:

...telling parents to 'slow down' resulted in shorter and simpler utterances in conjunction with a reduced rate of speech as well as increased latency of turn taking. Telling parents to 'slow down and use simpler language' drastically altered parent–child interactions in many cases, led to parental problems in formulating conversationally adequate speech, and prompted children to interrupt them frequently to complete their utterances. On a more casual level of analysis, the 'quality' of the interactions of those parents who had been told to make changes in both rate and complexity suffered. Parents stuck to 'safe' topics, short yes/no questions, and talked less. (p. 245)

Ratner is aware that more research needs to be done in this area but is sufficiently confident in her results to assert that advice to parents concerning their speech production may not be without harmful side-effects. She concludes that:

...carrying out dynamic and caring conversations with a child in a genuine manner may be quite difficult, if not impossible, when one is trying to adjust communicative behaviour to conform to rate, length and complexity guide-lines. (p. 245)

We may conjecture that many of these parents are able spontaneously to modify their rate of speech and level of linguistic complexity when they do so as a result of their particular interpretation of a situation or of a listener's need. It may be that asking them consciously to change their way of speaking puts them in an impossible, paradoxical situation of the 'be spontaneous' sort. That is, we want them to remain 'natural' while doing something that does not come naturally. Ratner is not saying parents should never be encouraged to modify their speech to better suit the child's current needs but is rather warning us to think carefully before we give such advice and to consider the possible consequences. It may also be important to suggest the modification of only one aspect of speaking and to evaluate the effects of this because, if Ratner's findings have a general applicability, then modification in one dimension will have a knock-on effect. This research also highlights the need to evaluate exactly what the changes are that we set in motion, so that we have a clearer idea of what it is that is making a difference.

There is another question raised by the popular suggestion that parents should reduce linguistic pressure by simplifying their own language, which concerns why this might be necessary. When parents quite obviously have very high expectations for their child's expressive language then assistance in communicating at a level appropriate to the child's language age makes sense. However, 'although stuttering may interact in theoretically and clinically interesting ways with language task demands, the condition of stuttering cannot be clearly linked to underlying deficiencies in language knowledge or to evidently atypical patterns of language performance' (Ratner, 1995a, p. 34).

There might be a sub-group of disfluent children who have other language difficulties, as was suggested by Van Riper in his developmental tracks (1982) but, when grouped together, there is little evidence to support the idea that children who stutter have significant language problems (Nippold, 1990). More research is needed to explore the relationship between various language tasks and stuttering if we are to be able effectively to remediate the subtle language difficulties of the group at risk. For the rest, there is a need to ensure that if reduction in linguistic complexity seems beneficial, then, as therapy develops, the child is helped to deal with language in everyday contexts. Language in context is often complex not just in the linguistic sense but because so many different factors are involved.

The idea of toughening up or reducing sensitivity to potentially disruptive stimuli is considered by Webster (1993) in his discussion of possible underlying factors. His research into brain function as suggested by performance in finger-tapping tasks has led him to postulate the idea of a 'Fragile Speech Motor Control System' (p. 101) in some adults who stutter. Webster thinks that for some at least this is a permanent fragility and that one way to minimise its effects might be to make automatic, as far as possible, the content of speech at times when the control system is most likely to be overloaded. In this way the speaker has more chance of being able to direct his or her attention towards the voluntary control of their speech mechanism. For example, a child who finds it stressful introducing himself may benefit from repeated rehearsal of how he will do this so that he can concentrate on easy onset and reduced rate while introducing himself. This is not without problems, however, as many people who stutter spend a lot of time in private rehearsal of feared speaking, only to find that when the time comes they cannot say what they have planned. Webster acknowledges the importance of desensitisation work and it may be that a certain level of confidence is necessary in order for the rehearsal to be a positive experience. Although Webster's work is with adults we must assume that the underlying problem was present in childhood and that we should strive to recognise this particular sub-group of children who have a fragile speech motor control system. Reduction in rate of parental speech and consequently also of linguistic complexity could have a positive effect, whether the underlying difficulty is motor speech or psycholinguistic in origin.

Reducing the Number of Questions Asked of the Child

Reduction in parental questions has already been mentioned with reference to the approaches described above and is also to be found in Irwin's (1988) book for parents. The presumed negative effect of asking questions was investigated by Weiss and Zebrowski (1991, 1992) in their study of responses compared with assertions. Although their sample was small, had a big age range and different levels of stuttering severity their results were sufficiently at odds with current wisdom to warrant further study. They found that the parents of stutterers do not produce more requests than do parents of non-stutterers and that 'children's disfluencies are overwhelming more likely to occur in assertive utterances, not in response to parents' requests' (Weiss, 1993, p. 221).

In addition they found that increased length and complexity seemed more likely to precipitate disfluencies regardless of whether the child's utterance was classed as a response or an assertion. There was a trend for parents to prefer lower level demands and for the children to be more disfluent in response to higher level demands (Weiss and Zebrowski, 1992). This finding supports the underlying rationale of the Stocker Probe Technique and perhaps, in time, a more reliable assessment of level of demand will evolve from further research of this type.

This research puts questions very much back on the families' agenda although some care would need to be taken regarding the level of demand inherent in different types of request if facilitation of fluency is the aim. Questions containing a forced alternative, such as 'Do you want chips or mash?', are probably the easiest, and open-ended requests – for example, to make up a story – the hardest (Stocker, 1980). There is some interesting work to be done in the area of demand but in the meantime it may be more useful to explore the parents' beliefs about how they should talk with their children and help them sort out the types of conversations that are relatively easy for a child from those that are difficult. For example, parents who believe that they must teach their child new words are likely habitually to extend the child's utterances which may interfere with following the child's lead. Guiding parents to tune into their child's wavelength and so talk about the things that the child is attending to in ways sympathetic to the child's level of development may be a better therapy option than telling them to reduce questions, which may have a negative effect on their interactions and the child's language development. The therapist is making a choice between first- and second-order changes, as discussed in the previous chapter.

Fluency Training vs Reducing Severity of Stuttering Behaviour

There is limited research that can be called upon to assist the therapist in making choices about one approach in preference to another. It was suggested at the beginning of the chapter that selection might be influenced by the hypotheses the therapist formulates regarding the underlying causal and maintaining factors. Therapy choices might also be influenced by the theoretical position of the therapist. For example, if one takes Webster's position then the child will need to be helped to find ways to compensate for 'the fragile speech motor control system' and the parents may need to be particularly careful to avoid putting undue extra pressure on the child. Tiredness, over-excitement and poor health may all reduce the child's ability to deal with his underlying problem. Verbal demands that require complex and quick responses are likely to be difficult. Fluency training along the lines of Meyers and Woodford's approach discussed earlier may well help the child to develop greater control in situations of gradually increasing complexity. There are also activity books, for example *Easy Does It* (Heinze and Johnson, 1985) and *Fluency at your Fingertips* (Ridge and Ray, 1991) that can be used in different ways by the therapist wanting to extend fluent speech.

Alternatively, the therapist might agree with Van Riper's (1990) ideas concerning a relatively short-term inconsistency in the development of all the areas required for fluent expressive speech and language. This view might lead the therapist to work on the environmental factors considered important if stuttering speech is not to develop into a stutter and the child become labelled as a stutterer (Perkins, 1992). Where the child is beginning to show signs of struggle and awarenes, open discussion about speaking can be helpful in reducing negative feelings. When parents can show their confidence in the child there is less risk that the child will interpret her disfluency as something bad and to be avoided.

It is of course possible that very different beliefs about stuttering might lead to the same therapeutic activities. If we consider a child who is fearful of introductions then this could lead to role play of such situations but with different aims depending upon theoretical rationale. For example, the aim could be to make the speech more automatic in line with Webster's thinking, or to find alternative ways of construing and hence behaving if the therapist took a personal construct view of stuttering (Hayhow and Levy, 1989) or to develop social skills if the therapist believed that stuttering children have poor social skills that need to be improved if fluency improvements are to be maintained (Rustin, 1987). In these three instances the therapy tasks would be approached in different ways and the evaluation of the child's performance would probably be done differently but it would be very hard to find support for any of the theoretical models simply by looking at therapy outcome. Perhaps this is why so many therapists end up taking a pragmatic and eclectic approach to stuttering. However interesting the theories regarding cause and maintenance, in the end what really matters is whether or not people respond positively to therapy. In addition, if we examine therapy evaluation data for speak more fluently vs stutter more fluently programmes for children there are so many other things being done that the role of direct speech work in final outcome is impossible to assess independently. Rustin (1984) attempted to tease out the effects of fluency training with and without social skills training in adolescents and found the combined therapy more effective than speech work alone. With young children it is more difficult to separate treatment effects, especially as now there is a general consensus that parents have an important role in therapy so we are not in a position to deprive some parents of therapy whilst we evaluate different speech techniques.

Working with Teachers

There is American literature for the school-based therapist but it does not readily translate into the therapy context here. There is very little literature on work with teachers in relation to stuttering in the UK, so therapists are often left to find out what they can do in their own particular circumstances. There are some general principles, however, that can be discussed.

It is generally accepted that teachers have had a difficult few years with apparently ever-increasing demands and an undermining of the status that they once enjoyed as a profession. The job of a speech and language therapist must seem a pretty soft option to many teachers and any suggestions from us that they should do extra work on behalf of the disfluent child may be too much to ask. In the author's experience many teachers suffer uncertainties and worries similar to those of parents when they first have to deal with a child who stutters. They want to do what is best for the child and are fearful of making things worse, they feel ignorant about stuttering and de-skilled when they fail to help the child speak more fluently. If it is a teacher who has referred the child for therapy then we can be fairly sure the stuttering is getting in the way of the child's relationships in school, possibly only with the teacher or maybe with peers as well.

The teacher is likely to require information about stuttering and also the opportunity to talk about any concerns with day-to-day handling. As with the parents, a list of do's and don'ts can increase anxiety and the feelings of being de-skilled, although many find leaflets such as the one published by the Association for Stammerers helpful. An increase in understanding, a feeling of confidence that they can do what is best for the child and a sense of security from the knowledge that they can talk about talking to the child can do much to facilitate a supportive atmosphere. Understanding the importance of providing the child with communication experiences and knowing how to manipulate the content and environment to increase the child's chances of success can help the teacher in daily management of the child. Meetings with the parents, older child, teacher and therapist can be organised so that there is a feeling of partnership facilitating a mutual exchange of relevant knowledge and expertise. It can be extremely helpful to the therapist to learn about the child's progress in school, particularly in respect of reading and spelling. If the child has problems in these areas then a further investigation of language and phonological skills may be appropriate (Klein, 1991).

As children get older they need to be involved in working out strategies to cope with problems and to feel that they have some control over the demands that will be made for verbal performance. So many adults remember feelings of fear, panic and helplessness as they sat waiting for their turn to speak. Often they would be so preoccupied with their fears that they would be unable to attend to the lesson prior to their turn and feel so ashamed after speaking that they were still unable to concentrate. Some teachers, out of their concern for the child, would apparently make the decision not to ask the stuttering child to speak. However, if the child was not informed of this decision they would still suffer the agonies of waiting a turn and yet never have the chance to prove to themselves that they could do it. Breaking the conspiracy of silence and helping the children and all those directly concerned with them to be open and optimistic about stuttering is an important first step in therapy. Trying to ensure that fluent speaking does not become the most important criterion for judging personal value is an important therapy aim and one that both teachers and parents can help with. Providing opportunities for the child to develop in as many areas as possible and encouraging an understanding of others can do much to help keep problems with speaking in proportion.

Children with Concomitant Language or Phonological Difficulties

Very little has been written about children with concomitant speech and language problems and yet research suggests that such children should make up a sizeable sub-group of the stuttering population. Therapy decisions concerning whether to work on, for example, fluency and then phonology or whether to attempt to integrate the different areas is well discussed by Ratner (1995b). The therapist will need to take account of the effect that the specific production demands may have on the child's fluency and also consider how fluency can be facilitated while working on production. In particular, developing ways of giving feedback that will not lead the child to undue self-awareness or criticism seems important. It may be difficult for parents to cope with increases in disfluency following apparent strides in language development; it may seem that the child is in an endless process of two steps forward and one step back. It is likely that children who have problems with several areas of speech and language development are particularly at risk. They are likely to experience more frequent disfluency and also the disfluency may last for a longer period of time than in those disfluent children who have normal language skills. If verbal communication is often frustrating for the child and his conversation partners then there is an available context in which negative attitudes can develop. Encouraging confidence and self-esteem would seem particularly important for such a child and the parents may also need extra support and guidance.

One conclusion that we can draw from the research and efficacy studies is that we must not lose touch with our creativity as therapists. There is no one way to treat children who stutter and if we try to force a child into a particular therapy model we may fail to help, or worse, by repeated failures, may encourage a belief that there is no help for the person who stutters. Similarly there is no right way of working with parents and we must take time to listen to their views and modify our approach to suit them. The last 20 years have seen many changes in speech and language therapy; it is a developing field and progress in the understanding and therapy of any of the developmental problems may well have implications for disfluency. Working with stuttering is challenging and offers the therapist a context for continued development. If we can convey this interest and commitment to developing our understanding of the problem then at least our disfluent clients will feel valued. If the child and parents can also take this view then they are more likely to be able to find ways of dealing with the problems that they encounter in their everyday lives. When therapists or parents feel that their behaviour is governed by lists of things they should and should not do they are likely to find stuttering frustrating and attempts to help the child may well prove unsuccessful. If we engage the parents actively in therapy so that they are free to comment on what we say and do then we should avoid giving advice that we later find is contradicted in the literature. When parents are encouraged to experiment carefully with change, we also reduce the risk of inflicting artificial communication patterns on the family that may in the long run do more harm than good.

References

Bateson, G. (1972). *Steps to an Ecology of Mind*. New York: Ballantine Books.

Botterill, W., Kelman, E. and Rustin, L. (1991). Parents and their pre-school stuttering child. In: L. Rustin (Ed.), *Parents, Families and the Stuttering Child*. Leicester: Far Communication Disorders.

Cunningham, C. and Davis, H. (1985). *Working with Parents: Frameworks for Collaboration*. Milton Keynes: Open University Press

Egan, G. (1986). *The Skilled Helper*. Monterey, CA: Brooks/Cole.

Gregory, H. (1979). Controversial issues: statements and review of the literature. In: H. Gregory (Ed.), *Controversies about Stuttering Therapy*. Baltimore: University Park Press.

Gregory, H. and Hill, D. (1980). Stuttering therapy for children. *Seminars in Speech Language and Hearing* 4, 351–364.

Hayhow, R. and Levy, C. (1989). *Working with Stuttering: A Personal Construct Approach*. Bicester, Oxon: Winslow Press

Heinze, B. and Johnson, K. (1985). *Easy Does it: Fluency Activities for [1] Young Children and [2] School-aged Stutterers*. Illinois: Lingui Systems.

Howell and Dean (1991). *Treating Phonological Disorders in Children: Metaphon – Theory to Practice*. Leicester: Far Communication Disorders.

Ingham, R. (1985). Stuttering treatment outcome evaluation: closing the credibility gap. *Seminars in Speech & Language* 6(2), 105–123.

Irwin, A. (1988). *Stammering in Young Children*. London: Association for Stammerers.

Klein, H. (1991). Stuttering: complex linguistic difficulties in adolescents. *Human Communication* 1(1).

Mater, C. (1993). The neural basis of language. In: E. Boberg (Ed.), *Neuropsychology of Stuttering*. Canada: University of Alberta Press.

Meyers, S. and Woodford, L. (1991). *The Fluency Development System for Young Children*. Aurora, NY: United Educational Services.

Nippold, N. (1990). Concomitant speech and language disorders in stuttering children: a critique of the literature. *Journal of Speech and Hearing Disorders* 55, 51–60.

Perkins, W. (1992). *Stuttering Prevented*. London: Whurr Publishers

Peters, T. and Guitar. B, (1991). *Stuttering: An Integrated Approach*. Baltimore: Williams & Wilkins.

Ratner, N. Bernstein (1992). Measurable outcomes of instructions to modify parent–child interaction. *Journal of Speech and Hearing Research* 35, 14–20.

Ratner, N. Bernstein (1993). Parents, children and stuttering. *Seminars in Speech and Language* 14(3), 238–250.

Ratner, N. Bernstein (1995a). Language complexity and stuttering in children. *Topics in Language Disorders* 15(3), 32–47.

Ratner, N. Bernstein (1995b). Training the child who stutters with concomitant language or phonological impairment. *Language, Speech and Hearing Services in Schools* 26(2), 180–186.

Ridge, H. and Ray, B. (1991). *Fluency at your Fingertips – Pragmatic and Thematic Therapy Materials*. Arizona: Communication Skill Builders.

Riley, G. and Riley, J. (1984). A component model for treating stuttering in children. In: M. Peins (Ed.), *Contemporary Approaches in Stuttering Therapy*, (pp.123–171). Boston, MA: Little, Brown.

Rommel, D., Johannsen, H., Schulze, H. and Hage, A. (1993). Onset, development and maintenance of childhood stuttering: a five year longitudinal study – preliminary results. Paper presented at the Third Oxford Disfluency Conference.

Rustin, L. (1984). Intensive treatment models for adolescent stuttering: a comparison of social skills training and speech fluency techniques. Unpublished MPhil thesis, Leicester Polytechnic, UK.

Rustin, L. (1987). *Assessment and Therapy Programme for Disfluent Children*. Windsor: NFER Nelson.

Ryan, B. (1974). *Programmed Therapy of Stuttering in Children and Adults*. Springfield, IL: Charles C. Thomas.

Seider, R., Gladstein, K. and Kidd, K. (1983). Recovery and persistence of stuttering among relatives of stutterers. *Journal of Speech and Hearing Disorders* 48, 402–409.

Starkweather, W., Gottwald, S. and Halfond, M. (1990). *Stuttering Prevention: a Clinical Method*. Englewood Cliffs, NJ: Prentice-Hall.

Stocker, B. (1980). *The Stocker Probe Technique for Diagnosis and Treatment of Stuttering in Young Children*. Tulsa, OK: Modern Education Corporation.

Van Riper, C. (1982). *The Nature of Stuttering*, 2nd edn. Englewood Cliffs, NJ: Prentice-Hall.

Van Riper, C. (1990). Final thoughts about stuttering. *Journal of Fluency Disorders* **15**, 317–318.

Webster, W. (1993). Hurried hands and tangled tongues. In: E. Boberg (Ed.), *Neuropsychology of Stuttering*. Canada: University of Alberta Press.

Weiss, A. (1993). The pragmatic context of children's dysfluency, *Seminars in Speech and Language* **14**(3), 215–225.

Weiss, A. and Zebrowski, P. (1991). Patterns of assertiveness and responsiveness in parental interactions with stuttering and fluent children. *Journal of Fluency Disorders* **16**, 125–143.

Weiss, A. and Zebrowski, P. (1992). Disfluencies in the conversations of young children who stutter: some answers about questions. *Journal of Speech and Hearing Research* **35**, 1230–1238.

Yairi, E. (1982). Longitudinal studies of disfluencies in two year old children. *Journal of Speech and Hearing Research* **25**, 155–160.

Chapter 4
Covert Aspects Associated with the 'Stuttering Syndrome': Focus on Self-Esteem

KHURSHEED BAJINA

In working with people who stutter, I have rarely come across any individual who did not make some reference to 'confidence', or 'self-worth' or 'feeling stupid'. After a course of therapy, the letters and comments received from clients did not identify improvement in speech as the major feature. Comments usually included statements such as 'feeling better about myself', 'my life has changed', 'I have a new job and a new boyfriend'.

The main aim of the original study (Bajina, 1992) was to propose a reinforcement model (see Figure 4.1) encompassing the covert variables investigated in this study. Two subject groups, the experimental group comprising 28 adults who stuttered and a control group comprising 25 adults who did not stutter, were compared on four covert aspects. These were state anxiety, trait anxiety, self-esteem and attitudes to interpersonal communication. The relationships between these covert variables, as well as avoidance and expectation, were explored.

It is not within the scope of this chapter to discuss all the results of the original study. However, summary tables and a diagram of the proposed model have been included. The self-esteem variable will be the main focus, with some reference to the relationship between anxiety and self-esteem. In this study, use of the Rosenberg (1965) Self-esteem Scale confirmed the hypothesis that the experimental group had a significantly lower self-esteem score than the control group. A significant difference was also obtained for trait anxiety using a self-evaluation questionnaire (Spielberger, 1983), and the S24 questionnaire for attitudes to interpersonal communication (Andrews and Cutler, 1974).

When this study was undertaken on the covert aspects of stuttering, there were concerns that the variables were not measurable, and that was why so few researchers had examined these aspects of stuttering. One of the conclusions I have drawn about people who stutter is that the most relevant factors in the occurrence of stuttering are subjective to the

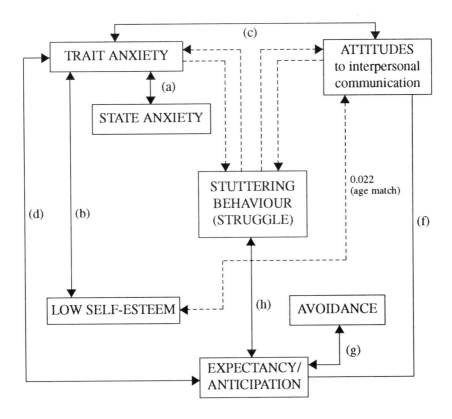

Figure 4.1 The Proposed Reinforcement Model (1992)

individual who stutters. Therefore it seemed pertinent to do a study based on personal inventories and questionnaires which would reveal the perceptions of the stutterers themselves.

These covert behaviours are not exclusive to adults who stutter. Anyone who has to go through life from early childhood with the life experiences of a stutterer would probably develop these covert behaviours in the same way, depending on their personality and coping strategies for life stresses and events in general. Most people have not experienced the repeated social rejections to which the mature stutterer has been exposed, nor have they 'felt the doubt that follows, the fear, and the growing negative expectancy toward others, with its ever accumulating denigration to the stutterer's self-concept' (Murphy, 1974).

The major insight developed by Cooper (1986), from a decade of research stimulated by Sheehan, was the irrelevance of noting the frequency of disfluencies in assessing stuttering. Cooper (1986) describes this as the 'frequency fallacy'. As a researcher with clinical experience, it appeared more important to discover the stutterer's own perspective on various covert aspects, as this seemed to be a more reliable measure of severity and allowed for the variability of the stuttering syndrome.

In addition to anxiety, the most common presenting attitudes of stutterers seem to be feelings of helplessness, victimisation and low self-esteem (Shames and Rubin, 1986). Hargie *et al.* (1987) define self-esteem as the worth which an individual bestows upon him- or herself and can range from feelings of love and acceptance to hate and rejection. In view of all the research identifying self-esteem, it was surprising that almost all of the literature reviewed on self-esteem made no reference to stuttering.

Williams (1988) reminds clinicians that there is no strong distinction between the evaluation of a stutterer's communication problem and his programme of therapy. Therefore, he recommends that clinicians discover as much as they can about how the stutterer came to be the kind of person he is today – the beliefs he has, his attitudes about himself, contrasted with attitudes and beliefs that create pride, strength, purpose and happiness.

Craig (1990) concurs with Williams's (1988) view that stutterers would be neurotic, insensitive or unaware of what is going on around them if they were as socially well adjusted as non-stutterers. Craig surmises that 'people who have had problems communicating and interacting with others most of their lives, may come to perceive the world in a more hostile light than someone who does not stutter, and who is of the same age, sex and occupation'.

Van Riper (1974) proposed that 'stuttering is not just a speech impairment, it is an impediment in social living'. Curlee (1984) reports, 'it has been in my clinical experience that adults [stutterers] readily report feelings, attitudes and beliefs that seem to interfere with their ability to cope satisfactorily with many of life's experiences that involve inter-personal communication...and may foster self-defeating behaviour'.

Michener *et al.* (1986) indicate three major sources of self-esteem: family experience, performance feedback and social comparison. Parent–child relationships are important for the development of self-esteem. Children with higher self-esteem exhibit more self-confidence, competence and self-control and they are likely to elicit responses from their parents that further promote self-esteem. Parents' responses to their children continue to have effects in adult life.

On a recent intensive course for adult stutterers, this view was illustrated by P.H.'s father who stated that 'P.H. is not so good at things. His 12-year-old brother is good at everything.' P.H. was unable to accept praise and reinforcement on the course. He would look away and look uncomfortable when given any positive feedback. P.H. revealed a bright humour and wit as the course progressed, which had obviously not been appreciated at home.

Campbell (1990) notes that the area in which self-esteem appears to exert especially powerful effects occurs in individual reactions to self-relevant feedback or information. Campbell suggests that low self-esteem people have poorly articulated notions of who or what they are. Feelings of self-worth are thought to vary over time and roles, and this variation is a common feature of stuttering.

There is a social expectation that fluency is the norm. People who stutter have to integrate both educationally and socio-economically in a predominantly fluent society. Because of prejudice and ignorance, a minority group is likely to see a negative image of themselves reflected in the appraisal of others (Campbell, 1990). With this in mind, the psychological, social and environmental factors associated with having a stutter cannot be ignored.

Michener *et al.* (1986) refer to the negative self-image of a minority group. If, because of prejudice, minority groups see a negative image of themselves in other's appraisals, then they will interpret their performances and achievements as evidence of their basic lack of worth and competence. Clients have often reported feelings of being different, feeling isolated, not knowing of others who stutter, as well as feeling abnormal.

By definition, stutterers are not only a minority group, but would also be considered abnormal ('away from the norm'; Atkinson *et al.,* 1983). Behaviour is abnormal if it is maladaptive, or if it has an adverse effect on the individual or society. Atkinson asserts that feelings of worthlessness, alienation and lack of acceptance are prevalent among individuals who are diagnosed as abnormal.

Our everyday successes and failures influence self-esteem by providing us with frequent feedback about the quality of our performances (Michener *et al.,* 1986). Social comparison is crucial to self-esteem because our feelings of competence depend in large part on the comparisons which we and others make. All techniques for protecting self-esteem portray human beings as active processors of social events (Michener et al., 1986). Stutterers often report that they have to protect themselves, and often avoid social participation for reasons of self-preservation.

An interesting study by Attanasio (1987) investigated the relationship between Lewis Carroll's stuttering, his use of nonsense, oral aggression and his treatment of communication failure in *Alice's Adventure's in Wonderland* and *Through the Looking Glass*. It is held by students of Lewis Carroll's work that the dodo is considered to be the (part-word) repetition of Carroll's real surname, Dodgson. Skinner (1971) remarks that it is interesting to recall the symbol of the dodo bird which is stupid, ineffective and aimless.

Wallen (1959), cited in Fransella (1972), differentiated stutterers from non-stutterers by showing stutterers to be less independent, more lacking in emotional control, less self-accepting and more self-rejecting. Fiedler and Wepman (1951), Fransella (1968), Kalinowski *et al.* (1987) found no significant difference in self-description between stutterers and non-stutterers. However, the stuttering subjects did tend to perceive the normal speaking population as superior to themselves.

Sheehan (1986) infers that the occurrence of stuttering is a function of how the stutterer feels about himself and especially about himself as a speaker. Sheehan's studies provided support for the theory of approach avoidance, for it became apparent that 80% of stutterers who recover, virtually unaided, attribute their success to their determination to confront and approach stuttering, to accept the role of stutterer and to build up self-esteem (Sheehan *et al.,* 1962, Sheehan and Martyn, 1966). Another concept put forward by Sheehan is the 'giant in chains' effect. When stutterers face their fear of stuttering and are open about it, its ego-protective function is removed.

The lower a person's self-esteem, the more likely he is to report experiencing various physiological indicators of anxiety (Rosenberg, 1965). Stutterers often report having 'sweaty palms' and shortness of breath in situations requiring inter-personal communication. Fromm-Reichman, cited in Rosenberg (1965), has suggested that anxiety is manifested by (among other factors) a feeling of uncertainty and helplessness, and a blocking of communication. According to Horney, cited in Rosenberg (1965), anxiety tends to generate low self-esteem.

Rosenberg considers four factors associated with low self-esteem which may be expected to create anxiety:

1. instability of self-image;
2. the presenting self;
3. vulnerability;
4. feelings of isolation.

Rosenberg suggests that control of these factors will decrease relationships of self-esteem to anxiety.

Another factor which may contribute to the association between self-esteem and anxiety is the tendency for people with low self-esteem to present a false front or face to the world. The false front is thought to be a coping mechanism. S.S. claimed, 'I'm fed up with covering up and putting on a front'. S.S. was a covert stutterer who has spent most of his life avoiding words, and putting himself across as a fluent speaker. C.K. had never discussed her stutter with her boyfriend of two years who assured the researcher, 'she doesn't stammer' when they both attended the initial assessment. Putting on this front is in itself anxiety-provoking, as putting on an act tends to be a strain. A second source of tension lies in the possibility that one will make a false step, reveal some inconsistency, or let the guise slip.

Schulz and Hanusa (1988) note that after a failure experience, individuals expect to do poorly and, in effect, do poorly on purpose in order to down-play the significance of their anticipated poor showing. Rubin (1986) refers to this as the self-fulfilling prophesy. Stutterer D.A. invited rejection by her behaviour, as this is what she expected. By not trying, subjects have a readily available unstable attribution for poor performance and, therefore, avoid any further threats to self-esteem. In a Kellyan sense this would compare with the 'hostility' felt when one's core constructs are threatened (Kelly, 1955, cited in Fransella, 1972).

Since the outcomes of ongoing actions are often fed back as ambiguous information, they are generally open to a number of possible interpretations (Spielberger and Sarason, 1988). Thus, individuals can develop a bias of attributing failure to their own actions. It is often very difficult for a stutterer to reframe a situation in a positive light. They will often interpret listener reactions in a negative way in the absence of any evidence.

Dunkel-Schetter *et al.* (1987) reviewed the six most widely used coping measures using 'The Ways of Coping Inventory'. Two of these were wishful thinking (engaging in fantasies about escaping or avoiding the situation), and self-blame. These appear to be particular characteristics of people high in trait anxiety (McCrae and Costa, 1986). It is possible that the covert behaviours, beliefs and attitudes learned by stutterers over time may be a natural process developed in order to cope with stuttering in a social context, and to preserve self-esteem as far as possible.

The self-esteem questionnaire used in the study (Rosenberg, 1965) investigates respect for self and other areas of self-worth. Rosenberg measured self-esteem using a 10-item Guttman scale, which has satisfactory reproducibility and scalability. The following practical and theoretical considerations were taken into account when selecting this scale:

1. ease of administration;
2. economy of time;
3. unidimensionality: subjects were required to rank people along a single continuum from those who had very high to those with very low self-esteem.

The difference between the experimental and control groups on the self-esteem variable was highly significant at a 0.001 level.

Michener *et al.* (1986) defined self-esteem as the evaluative component of the self-concept. From this result one concludes that stutterers as a group have a more negative self-concept than non-stutterers. Campbell (1990) noted that self-esteem exerts powerful effects with respect to people's reaction to self-relevant feedback or information. Clinical experience suggests that stutterers appear to expect the worst reactions based on past experience. They often predict that people judge them as being stupid and unable to do things fluent people can do. Covert stutterers frequently report that they have to hide the fact that they stutter and so they live a lie.

Michener *et al.* (1986) also state that people with low self-esteem tend to be socially anxious, feel less positively towards others and are easily hurt by criticism.

The four final items on the self-esteem scale look at self-worth (i.e. feelings towards self, which is a definition of self-esteem), whereas the first five items on the scale look at perceived comparisons between self and others on general ability. It appears that, from the stutterer's own perspective, they have very little respect for themselves and often feel useless, like the dodo in Carroll's *Alice in Wonderland* (Attanasio, 1987). However, they do see themselves as having good qualities and abilities equal to those of others. Perhaps the difference in responses between the former and latter items is the stutterer's perceived role. It is possible that when he considers 'self' the stuttering role predominates.

If all techniques for protecting self-esteem portray human beings as active processors (Michener *et al.*, 1986), and if various avoidance strategies are techniques used by stutterers, then this would account for why the desensitisation process and avoidance reduction are so painful. In therapy, clinicians are attempting to pull down the stutterer's own defence mechanism built up over time to protect his or her self-esteem.

If stutterers, as has been found in this study, are different from the 'norm' in their attitudes and self-esteem and feel abnormal, then, as Atkinson *et al.* (1983) assert, feelings of worthlessness and alienation will be prevalent. Stutterers often report feelings of isolation. M.C. reported that she had never met another female stutterer and had never before realised there were people with her problems anywhere. She felt less isolated and alienated as she developed self-worth which she called 'respect for herself' and 'self-confidence'. In the researcher's experience as a clinician, building self-worth and challenging negative statements about self as part of the overall approach have been effective. As Murphy (1974) surmises, feelings of self-worth may be the key to enhancing personal relationships.

A significant relationship was found between state and trait anxiety, even though there was no significant difference found between the experimental and control groups on state anxiety (see Table 4.1).

This result supports the contention that the higher the anxiety trait, the more probable it is that the individual will experience more intense elevations in state anxiety in threatening situations (Endler and Edwards, 1982, cited in Bolger, 1990; Spielberger *et al.*, 1983). This would account for the intensified expectation of failure and avoidance of perceived anxiety-provoking situations, further reinforcing low self-esteem.

This result would suggest that stutterers do tend to interpret a wider range of situations as dangerous and threatening. This was borne out by the fact that the experimental group were able to name several anxiety-

Table 1 Correlations: 28 Subjects (experimental group only)

	State	Trait
State	$r = 1.0000$	$r = 0.5283$
	(28)	(28)
	$P = .*$	$P = .002$
	sig.	sig.
Trait	$r = 0.5283$	$r = 1.0000$
	(28)	(28)
	$P = .002$	$P = .*$
	sig.	sig.

There is a significant relationship between state and trait anxiety at the $P < 0.001$ level of significance $r = 0.5283$ $p = 0.002$

provoking situations involving communication without giving it much thought, whereas the control group often found it difficult to identify a single such situation, as though they had never thought about it.

So what is the danger and threat of the situation involving inter-personal communication for the stutterer? Stutterers often report that they fear stuttering in these situations. When asked why, they usually make a response relating to the listener's reaction. They feel embarrassed and frustrated. They report that people 'smile' in a derogatory way, or tease or even laugh outright. These issues all relate to denigration of self-esteem.

When children begin to develop a construct sub-system about speech, this is usually due to observing the reactions of parents, family and teachers to them speaking. When they are asked to 'say it again' or 'slow down and take a breath', it is thought that they start thinking they are doing something wrong from a very early stage. This inevitably affects self-esteem. Anxiety in speaking situations would be a natural consequence.

A high correlational relationship was found between trait anxiety and self-esteem. Thus the higher the trait anxiety the lower the self-esteem. This result concurs with the view of Rosenberg (1965) who suggests that the lower a person's self-esteem, the more likely he is to report experiencing various manifestations of anxiety (see Table 4.2).

Rosenberg's 'false front' hypothesis regarding the association between self-esteem and anxiety was also supported by these results. It might have been useful to divide the group of stutterers into more 'covert' and more 'overt' to see if the relationship between anxiety and self-esteem was stronger for stutterers whose stutter manifested itself more covertly, where they were putting on a false front. The implications of the study for treatment and management are considered in a subsequent chapter.

Table 2 Correlations: 28 Subjects (experimental group only)

	State	Trait
Trait	r = 1.0000	r = 0.4766
	(28)	(28)
	P = .*	P = .005
	sig.	sig.
Self-esteem	r = 0.4766	r = 1.0000
	(28)	(28)
	P = .005	P = .*
	sig.	sig.

There is a significant relationship between trait and self-esteem at the $P < 0.001$ level of significance $r = 0.4766$ $p = 0.005$

References

Andrews, G. and Cutler, J. (1974). Stuttering therapy: the relation between changes in symptom level and attitudes. *Journal of Speech and Hearing Disorders* **39**, 312–319.

Atkinson, R.L., Atkinson, R.C. and Hilgard, E.R. (1983). *Introduction to Psychology*, 8th edn. New York: Harcourt Brace Jovanovich.

Attanasio, J.S. (1987). The DoDo was Lewis Carroll: reflections and speculations. *Journal of Fluency Disorders* **12**, 107–118.

Bajina, K. (1992) An Investigation of the Covert Aspects Associated with the Stuttering Syndrome—A Reinforcement Model.

Bolger (1990) Coping as a personality process: A prospective study. *Journal of Personality and Social Psychology* **59**(3), 525–537.

Campbell, J.D. (1990). Self-esteem and the clarity of the self-concept. *Journal of Personality and Social Psychology* **59**(3), 538–549.

Cooper, E.B. (1986). Joseph G. Sheehan's contributions: an eagle soars. *Journal of Fluency Disorders* **11**, 175–182.

Craig, A. (1990). An investigation into the relationship between anxiety and stuttering. *Journal of Speech and Hearing Disorders* **55**, 290–294.

Curlee, R.S. (1984) Stuttering disorders: An overview. In: Costello, J.M. (Ed.), Speech Disorders in Children: Recent Advances. San Diego: College Hill.

Dunkel-Schetter, C., Folkman, S. and Lazarus, R. (1987). Correlates of social support receipt. *Journal of Personality and Social Psychology* **53**(1), 71–80.

Fiedler and Wepman (1951) An exploratory investigation of the self-concept of stutterers. *Journal of Speech and Hearing Disorders* **16**, 110–114.

Fransella, F. (1970). Stuttering: not a symptom but a way of life. *British Journal of Disorders of Communication* **5**, 20–29.

Fransella, F. (1972). *Personal Change and Reconstruction*. London and New York: Academic Press.

Hargie, O., Saunders, C. and Dickson, D. (1987). *Social Skills in Interpersonal Communication*. London: Croom Helm.

Kalinowski, J.S., Lerman, J.W. and Watt, J. (1987). A preliminary examination of the perceptions of self and others in stutterers and nonstutterers. *Journal of Fluency Disorders* **12**, 317–331.

Kelly, G.A. (1955). *The Psychology of Personal Constructs*. New York: Norton.

McRae, R.R. and Costa, P.T. (1986). Personality, coping and coping effectiveness in an adult sample. *Journal of Personality* **54**, 385–405.

Michener, H.A., DeLamater, J.D. and Schwartz, S.H. (1986). *Social Psychology*. New York: Harcourt Brace Jovanovich.

Murphy, A. (1974). Feelings and attitudes. In: Starkweather, C.W. (Ed.), *Therapy for Stutterers*, pp. 87–104. Speech Foundation of America Publication No. 10.

Rosenberg, M. (1965). When dissonance fails: On eliminating evaluation apprehension from attitude measurement. *Journal of Personality and Social Psychology* **1**(1), 28–42.

Rubin, H. (1986). Cognitive therapy (postscript). In: Shames, G.H. and Rubin, H., *Stuttering Then and Now*. Seattle: Merrill.

Schulz, R. and Hartman Hanusa, (1988). Information seeking, self-esteem and helplessness. In: Abramson, L.Y., *Social Cognition and Clinical Psychology*, Ch. 4. New York: Guildford.

Shames, G.H. and Rubin, F. (1986). *Stuttering Then and Now*. Seattle: Merrill.

Sheehan, J.G., Cortese, P. and Hadley, R. (1962). Guilt, shame and tension in graphic projections of stuttering. *Journal of Speech and Hearing Disorders* **6**, 249–254.

Sheehan, J.G. and Martyn, M.M. (1966). Spontaneous recovery from stuttering. *Journal of Speech and Hearing Research* **9**, 121–135.

Sheehan, V.M. (1986). Approach avoidance and anxiety reduction. In: Shames, G.H. and Rubin, H. *Stuttering Then and Now*. Seattle: Merrill.,

Spielberger, C.D. with Gorsuch, R.L., Lushene, R., Vagg, P.R. and Jacobs, G.A. (1983). *State–Trait Anxiety Inventory (Form Y) (Self-evaluation Questionnaire)*. Consulting Psychologists Press.

Van Riper, C. (1974). Modification of behaviour. In: Starkweather, C.W. (Ed.), *Therapy for Stutterers*. Speech Foundation of America Publication No. 10.

Wallen, V. (1959). A Q technique study of self-concepts of adolescent stutterers and non-stutterers. Unpublished PhD dissertation, Boston University.

Williams, D. (1988). *Stuttering Therapy: Prevention and Intervention with Children*, ed. J. Fraser. Speech Foundation of America Publication No. 20.

Chapter 5
Working with Adolescents

MAGGIE FAWCUS

Adolescence has traditionally been viewed as a period of storm and stress, and this has tended to be confirmed by media coverage of drug abuse, teenage pregnancies and increasing juvenile crime. In reality, of course, many adolescents pass through this stage to adulthood relatively unscathed. Adolescence has now come to be regarded as a transitional phase, a period of adjustment to physical and social change which may cause problems but is not by definition problematic.

For the adolescent who stammers, however, these changes, by their very nature, may cause additional difficulties which have not been encountered in childhood. If we are to meet the needs of the adolescent client, then we need to be cognisant of these potential areas of conflict, stress and low self-esteem. As Schwartz (1993) comments, 'adolescents as a group have some specific emotional concerns that also need to be addressed as part of a comprehensive therapy programme'. In spite of this, he observes that there is a paucity of literature available on specific approaches for this client group. Whilst we cannot, within the confines of this chapter, look at the theories of adolescent development which are emerging, we will look at some factors which seem to have particular relevance to an adolescent growing up with a stammer.

There is considerable variation in the age at which puberty occurs, and either early or late maturation can be a source of embarrassment. Blyth *et al.* (1983) found that being out of step in physical development with your peers has a more negative effect on boys than girls. This finding may have some implications for the boy who stammers, who already feels disadvantaged because of his disfluent speech, a fact which may be compounded by an early or late maturation.

Jackson and Bosma (1992) comment on the increase in the range of environments to which the adolescent is exposed. Where parental guidance or support is not available, the adolescent is having to fall back on his own resources. They go on to say that 'new situations and the demands they present are likely to encourage the development of additional personal resources and skills'. They observe, however, that the skills necessary for the appropriate social response may not have been developed and we can see that the shy adolescent can be disadvantaged in new situations which demand communication.

Damon (1983) and Hartup (1982), both cited by Coleman and Hendry (1990) found that an adolescent's conversational ability was related to socialisation and social acceptance. Coleman and Hendry went on to say, 'effective social interactions are important for adjustment, as they are necessary for an adolescent to make friends, become part of a peer group, develop social relationships, and become an independent, socially competent individual'. Even more pertinent for the adolescent who stutters is Coleman and Hendry's statement that telephoning and being telephoned are indices of status, popularity and peer group affiliation and therefore contribute to an adolescent's self-esteem. For the person who stutters and regards using the telephone as a situation to be feared and avoided, this may be a potent factor in limiting social interaction.

With verbal communication playing such an important part in the development of social relationships, the person who stutters is clearly at a disadvantage. Brooks-Gunn and Paikoff (1992) report on research that shows an increase in negative self-feelings, particularly during the first half of adolescence. It would seem reasonable to suppose that the adolescent who stutters would be more likely than most to share such feelings. Brennan (1982), cited by Coleman and Hendry, found that adolescents who described themselves as lonely, shy or socially anxious participated less often than their more sociable colleagues in peer activities (they dated less often, spent more time alone and participated in fewer extracurricular activities).

Adolescence is a transitional period from dependence to independence, and sometimes the bid for independence can bring about conflict with parents and teachers. 'Whilst freedom may at times appear the most exciting of goals', comment Coleman and Hendry (1990), 'there are moments when, in the harsh light of reality, independence and the necessity to fight one's own battles becomes a daunting prospect.' Adolescents still seek and need the support of concerned parents even whilst they are becoming increasingly involved with their peer group.

Newman and Newman (1976), cited by Coleman and Hendry, consider that the peer group is important in the development of a social identity and in providing supportive social relationships to aid the adolescent's withdrawal from emotional dependence on parents.

The adolescent is facing the challenge of changing roles, and these roles are going to place increasing demands on his ability to communicate, whether in talking with the opposite sex, coping with oral examinations or going for job interviews. To add to all this are the increasing uncertainties in finding employment. Coleman (1993) has written about the status ambiguity facing adolescents and comments that 'the feeling of not knowing where you stand, of not knowing exactly how you are going to be treated – as a child or as an adult – can be very difficult to cope with'.

An interesting pilot study by Rustin and Klein (1991) found that 53% of their 15 adolescent subjects obtained below-average scores on reading accuracy, expressive naming, receptive vocabulary and phonemic analysis and synthesis of single words. They commented: 'if stutterers present with subtle, sophisticated yet persistent and disabling high-order linguistic differences, these may extend to their pragmatic skills and may limit social interaction'. We know very little about school achievement in adolescents who stutter, but findings such as these imply that some of them may have additonal difficulties in coping with reading and other linguistic demands.

Whilst we have a wealth of clinical experience about how adolescents who stutter feel about themselves and their communicative abilities, there is a paucity of research into this area. None the less, research into adolescence in general gives us some useful guidelines in our management of the adolescent who stutters.

The Rationale for Group Therapy

We have already spoken of the importance of the peer group in the social development of adolescents, and it would therefore seem to make sense to involve those who stutter in their own peer group. It is not uncommon for children and adolescents who stutter to see themselves as totally unique in their dilemma, having never met anyone else who stutters. This may bring about a feeling of social isolation which is immediately alleviated by meeting peers who also stutter.

If positive change is to be brought about, it is important that the client, of whatever age, begins to feel good about his or her stutter. Meeting others who stutter, and the bonding that takes place in a supportive group setting, is the important beginning to this process. Group members are encouraged to become objective observers, to find out about their stutter by sharing experiences with other group members, and by carrying out real-life assignments.

Negative feelings of anxiety and embarassment, which adolescent boys in particular may normally find difficult to disclose, are aired and shared and found to be a problem for them all.

Much can be achieved in individual sessions, but the group situation is a powerful force for change. Lawson (1992) has written an interesting account of group work with adults, much of which is equally applicable to working with adolescents. 'Being liked, accepted, and finding one's identity in a group', say Coleman and Hendry (1990), 'are important at any age, but may be particularly crucial during adolescence.' In a group for adolescents who stutter we can try and ensure that each group member has that positive experience.

In the following pages we shall be describing and discussing the goals and activities which can be employed to achieve the sevenfold goals of our approach:

- reducing anxiety and embarrassment;
- reducing, and if possible, eliminating avoidance;
- achieving an acceptable and 'comfortable' level of non-fluency;
- eliminating those verbal or non-verbal behaviours (such as the use of excessive interjections and avoiding eye-contact) which interfere with effective communication;
- encouraging good communication skills;
- extending experience of communication situations and developing the linguistic and social skills necessary to tackle them successfully;
- increasing self-esteem.

Fluency-shaping Techniques

Our clients come to us seeking fluency, and it is tempting to offer them a technique which can enable them to experience immediate fluency. Many clients, however, have already been taught fluency-shaping techniques, and have either rejected them at the outset or found their effects were not lasting.

Nobody who is seriously involved in the management of stuttering can fail to have been caught up in the speak-more-fluently vs stutter-more-fluently controversy. Having worked with both approaches, I now have little doubt that we should not normally teach fluency techniques. This is not to say, however , that we are not concerned with modifying speech behaviour in the direction of normal. This will be discussed in a later section.

There seem to be some very good reasons why we should adopt a stutter-more-fluently approach: the first is a theoretical one. It seems fairly certain that anxiety about stuttering is fuelled by avoidance and, however overtly fluent a stutterer may be, he still often feels that he is walking the tightrope of fluent speech. This is an anxiety-provoking state of affairs, leading to still further avoidance at both the word and situation level, and to the maintenance of stuttering. When we advocate a technique such as slowed or prolonged speech we are in fact colluding with this avoidance. We are essentially teaching our clients to bypass the problem, and in so doing we do nothing to decrease his fear or embarrassment. We could even say that we are ensuring the maintenance of stuttering because we are not really addressing one crucial aspect of the problem. There is no doubt that in many cases the attitudes towards stuttering, whether they are labelled fear, anxiety, embarrassment, nervousness, self-consciousness or whatever, are more than half the problem, and encouraging stutterers to avoid blocking behaviour by using such techniques at best perpetuates the status quo.

There is a more serious side to the use of such fluency-shaping techniques: following an intensive course, the stutterer may experience a heady period of fluency. We know from clinical experience that these periods are frequently short-lived. Losing fluency after such a period is a demoralising experience, both for the therapist and the client, and also for the parents. They may feel guilty that they have failed to ensure that their child has maintained her fluency level. The client may lose faith in herself or in her therapist, or both. Everyone concerned is experiencing a feeling of failure to some extent or other.

There is one other point to be considered, and few therapists have not encountered this problem. Whilst the client may find that the technique effectively produces fluency, the technique may still be rejected as unnatural. Alternatively the client may appear to lack the motivation to make the necessary commitment to maintaining the technique. Maybe the stutterer is instinctively right in rejecting a technique with which he is not comfortable, and which can let him down so badly. We should certainly not sit in judgement over his apparent failure to carry out our prescription.

Sheehan (1975) has summed up the position on this question of fluency techniques succinctly and effectively. 'To make stutterers fluent in a sheltered environment is as meaningless as it is easy. The perceptive clinician soon learns what nearly every stutterer knows: that fluent intervals lead neither to a diminution of fear nor to a solution of the problem.'

Modifying Speech Behaviour

Changing speech behaviour demands a level of knowledge and self-awareness, which is also one of the most powerful tools in bringing about permanent change. This can occur not only in the overt behaviours which make up the stutter, but also in the whole infrastructure of attitudes.

The changes we want to make are long-lasting ones, which may be slower to achieve, but give the stutterer soundly based confidence in himself and his speech.

How do we bring about these changes? In the first place, rather than the sterile business of block-counting, we make a careful profile of the speech and other behaviours we wish to change. This is ideally carried out in the group, where group members may recognise behaviours in others which they themselves possess.

Group members are introduced to the idea that stuttering is a kind of formula: that it is not a unitary thing, but a galaxy of behaviours. Rather than 'getting rid of stuttering', a task which has always resulted in failure and even in a worsening of the stuttering (e.g. in attempts which have been made to hide or postpone stuttering), the stutterer is encouraged to have realistic goals of eliminating one or more of his stuttering behaviours.

The idea of a cluster of behaviours which combine to produce what we call stuttering can be a very useful one, as it allows us to tackle 'bits' of behaviour and therefore set goals which can be achieved. Furthermore, this is essentially a client-centred approach because everyone has their individual profile, which is quite unique to them, giving us a clear baseline from which to work. We must bear in mind that the attitudes – the avoidance behaviours, the anxieties and the embarrassments – are also all part of that galaxy.

These behaviours can be realised within the framework of Sheehan's 'iceberg', and this is a very good group activity in which to introduce the concept of overt and covert behaviours. As mentioned, covert feelings which a stutterer may be embarrassed to admit to become acceptable and normal within the group where these feelings are found to be shared. 'How I feel when I stammer/stutter' is a very useful brainstorming exercise to follow the profiling activity on overt behaviours.

We use the following formula:

Stutter = Core block + abnormal speech behaviours + abnormal non-verbal behaviours + avoidance + negative emotions (CB + ASB + ANVB + A + NE)

An individual profile might look like this:

Stutter = (silent laryngeal block) + (frequent use of back-tracking + interjection 'er') + (poor eye-contact + putting hand over mouth) + (avoidance of words, particularly beginning with /s/ + avoidance of the telephone and shopping) + (feel ashamed and feel angry when I stammer)

We can begin to break up the habitual pattern of stuttering by choosing one of these behaviours as a target for change, and each bit changed or eliminated leads to a reduction in the individual's stutter. In the case above we might start by encouraging eye-contact during the moment of stuttering, and by eliminating back-tracking.

This idea can be presented in a graphic two-dimensional way by presenting the client with a postcard, and asking him to write down his bits of abnormal behaviour on the postcard. He is told to give each item a different amount of space, in order to reflect the importance of the elements disrupting his speech behaviour. The postcard picture of the profile above would look something like this:

Looking away
when I stammer

Putting in 'um' before
a difficult word

Lowering my head when
I stammer

Banging my hand
on my leg

Taking in a gasp of breath
before a difficult word

He then selects the item of behaviour he wishes to modify or eliminate and cuts that piece out of the postcard, so that the dimension of stuttering is that bit less. This gives a small tangible goal, which is achievable. We find that it can be a very effective way of working towards what we call a 'comfortable' stutter.

Another way of getting rid of what we have termed 'rubbish' is to have a wastepaper basket (most younger clients are fully familiar with the wastebasket on the computer screen). The bit of behaviour being targeted is written down on a piece of paper, which is then screwed up and thrown very decisively into the waste-bin!

Finding that their habitual behaviours can be tackled in this way not only makes people who stutter aware of what they are doing, but also gives them a feeling of personal achievement. The aim is to 'whittle down' the behaviours which interfere with successful communication until one reaches the core block (which may also have changed during this process). One sometimes finds that when all the rubbish has been cleared away, there is little or nothing left. It is as if these behaviours have accrued round some imaginary 'black hole' which does not in fact exist.

The Core Block

The core block occurs because words are being approached in an abnormal way, often because the speaker has predicted that he will stammer on that word and therefore approaches it as if it were indeed 'difficult' . He is thus effectively ensuring that he blocks and therefore confirms his predictions about that sound or that word. However, prediction does not always seem to be involved, particularly where the client has very brief blocks. One gains the impression that these are habitual responses of which the speaker is sometimes barely aware. Both these cases will be discussed later in this section.

The core block can be remarkably impervious to attempts at change, and we then have to ask to what extent it interferes with effective communication, and to what extent the client is prepared to make the commitment to change. Clearly, all this will hinge quite heavily on the severity of the blocks and the client's level of concern or embarrassment about them. If the blocks are more severe, and not too frequent, then it is worth working to achieve more comfortable blocks with less struggle behaviour. Blocks occur because the speaker is employing too much pressure at some point in the vocal tract (e.g. between the lips) or at two points (e.g. at the level of the vocal folds and the alveolus). They may also occur because he is attempting to realise the sound with an abnormal articulatory posture (an actual example occurred where the speaker was attempting to say a word beginning with /s/ – the place where he lived – with a wide-open mouth). There is often a problem with inappropriate voicing, usually linked to over-tense closure of the vocal folds. So if we are to modify these blocks, the speaker needs to check the following:

Am I using the correct degree of pressure to enable this sound or word to come out?

Is the sound being made in the right place?

Am I using voice appropriately?

None of this can take place until the person begins to feel more comfortable about his stutter. If he is 'panicky' and embarrassed it is probably unrealistic to expect much in the way of modification.

We find it useful to make the client aware of the normal pressures and postures used in speech. Models or diagrams can show where sounds are made. We have an ancient pickled larynx which is a very popular way of making a group more aware of the voice mechanism! In addition to a very basic introduction to phonetics, we experiment with making sounds.

These activities include word games in which we pick a sound (e.g. /p/) and everyone in the group has to think of a word with that sound, or preferably two /p/ sounds (e.g. paper). These are tried out, first whispering to oneself to feel the small amount of pressure needed to produce the sound, and then aloud to the rest of the group. We look at where the sound is made and whether it is voiced or not.

Voicing is another aspect of speech which is studied in the group, encouraging everyone to feel what is going on in the larynx. The names of each group member are written on the board and we 'experiment' saying the names to find out which sounds are voiced or not, by placing a hand on the larynx. We try simulating laryngeal blocks, contrasting this with gentle voice onset. Experimenting, even block swapping, is very important in taking the feeling of helplessness out of stuttering, and demonstrating that these behaviours can be undertood and, more importantly, changed.

Generally speaking, this is as far as we go in teaching 'techniques'. We have regular 'block mod' sessions during an intensive course, to make sure everyone understands what is happening when they stammer and how they can change what is happening.

Fluency-shaping techniques are only 'on offer', as it were, when blocking is of very short duration, and it is then suggested that if the client is concerned about his blocks he can try speaking more slowly, using light contacts. This option is seldom taken up, and further illustrates how unrealistic it is to expect clients to maintain what they seem to view as an unnatural way of talking (however natural it can sound with practice).

Whilst the techniques described above are directed at the overt behaviours of stuttering, they are equally important in the whole process of attitude change. The person who stutters is already learning to become more objective and less emotional about his stutter as he observes it, studies it and discusses it with other people in a non-threatening and non-judgemental environment.

Avoidance and Assignments

Avoidance is a very sensitive indicator of the person's attitude to her stutter. It is a problem which is not always adequately addressed in therapy, but should always be an important area of focus in planning a therapy programme.

The effects of avoidance are insidious in maintaining word and situation fears. Because the reduction or elimination of avoidance can be a very threatening business, however, we need to present a clear rationale if we are to convince our clients of the need to work on avoidance.

Avoidance may be manifest at a number of different levels. At the microscopic level specific sounds or words are avoided, and many people who stutter become so adept at word avoidance that they are not always concious of doing it. They may develop a wealth of synonyms or strategies to meet their needs (such as presenting their card instead of giving their name when meeting new business associates). At the macroscopic level, avoidance may mean a reduction in what is said, to such an extent in some cases that only essential information is communicated, with none of the 'small talk' which most people enjoy.

In the middle, as it were, are the situations which are feared and avoided. Whilst there are a number of situations which are commonly avoided by most people who stutter, such as the telephone and shopping, each person's inventory of avoided situations has its unique aspects. It is therefore very important that we know what is avoided in attempting to deal with the problem. It is useful, once the situations have been listed, to place them in rank order. Although we may, after discussion with the client, decide to tackle the least feared and avoided situation, many clients cope well with starting much higher on their hierarchy list, particularly if an avoided situation is presenting problems socially or at school or work. This may be particularly true in using the telephone. Although this situation can cause considerable anxiety, tackling it early in therapy may give the client increased confidence.

The implications of eliminating avoidance are considerable. Avoidance is usually based on certain predictions that stuttering will occur if the speaker approaches the situation. Because the person who stutters is fearful that this will happen, particularly where he is uncertain of the audience reaction (e.g. speaking to strangers) he chooses to avoid that situation if he possibly can. Unfortunately, he does not therefore find out whether his predictions are correct. This is true not only for whether or not he will stutter, but more importantly for how the listener will react. In personal construct psychology terms, because he cannot predict events, he experiences anxiety.

In combating avoidance it would seem that the most important step is to help the speaker build up a store of experiences of listener reactions so that he may more reliably predict how people will behave if he does stutter. So the first assignment we should give a young person who stutters is the opportunity to observe audience reactions. Many non-fluent speakers make a hypothesis that the listener will react in an unfavourable way (such as laughing or walking away). This is seldom if ever put to the test, so we must give our clients the opportunity to test out their hypothesis. Here is a list of assignments designed to encourage this fact-finding exercise:

Ask a young lady the time.
Ask a young man the time.
Ask an older man the time.
Ask an older woman the time.
Ask a young lady the way to the nearest post office.
Ask a young man the way to the public library.
Ask an older woman where you can find a baker's shop.
Ask an older man the way to the nearest station.

The effects of carrying out these assignments are often quite profound, not only because the hypothesis is nearly always invalidated, but because the person who stutters is taking some important steps towards a more objective approach to his problem. Of course, occasional adverse reactions can occur, but these are normally of the over-helpful kind. Where adverse reactions do occur it is important to sit down and discuss them afterwards. The over-helpful reaction is often a rather clumsy way in which the listener tries to empathise with the speaker, and should be accepted as such. Where less helpful reactions are encountered, such as looking away, we must try and look at the possible reasons for them. This may be the point at which the client is encouraged to look at stuttering from another person's point of view; the listener may be equally embarrassed, for example, and this may well be the case when a socially inadequate young shop assistant laughs. The client needs to be aware that he can try and manipulate the situation to his advantage by trying to create a less threatening atmosphere for both himself and his listener. It may just be a matter of smiling before you start speaking or, more ambitiously, actually mentioning in a non-apologetic way that you stutter.

It is important to stress that the aim of assignments is not to be fluent. The person who stutters has tried that many times and failed. We do not want to add to the feeling of failure. This could, of course, be a good argument for using a fluency technique, but that would lose the whole point of an approach which is designed to take the fear out of stuttering. To be fluent would put the speaker on an emotional high, but we know from experience how fragile this thin layer of confidence is and, furthermore, it has not addressed the core problem of worrying how people might react if you stutter. Only by giving the person who stutters ample opportunity to find out how people really react, and moreover how he copes, can lasting changes be made in the negative feelings which surround the stutter.

It is certainly not essential to follow a strict hierarchy in carrying out a programme of assignments. It is usually wise to start with a number of the same assignments, such as asking between five and 10 people in the street if they can give you the time. In Kellyan terms this enables the client to start making the predictions which will reduce his anxiety about tackling this type of situation. On the principle that the bigger the investment made the more interest will be earned, we may encourage the client to go for a more demanding situation, such as an extended enquiry about a holiday in Spain in a travel agency. In making decisions about the kind of assignments to tackle, the clinician must be sensitive to the emotional robustness or otherwise of his or her client. It is essential, in this author's opinion, that early assignments are supervised. Not only does this enable the clinician to pick up the pieces if the assignment does go wrong but, perhaps more importantly, it enables her to give objective feedback on the client's performance. Early assignments can feel very threatening and the accompanying clinician can provide support and guidance where it is needed.

Debriefing sessions, either individually or in the group, should follow the assignments, so that performance can be discussed and evaluated. This is particularly important if the assignments have not gone well for any reason. Some people who stutter have a very negative view of their performance, and the therapist will need to feed back the positive apects to the client. The goal is to get the message across. Was this achieved, and if so, how effectively? Were there any behaviours, apart from stuttering, that interfered with effective communication? How could the situation be tackled on a future occasion?

Problem Solving

Adverse audience reactions, real, imagined or anticipated, are responsible for attempts to avoid, disguise or postpone the moment of stuttering. As already mentioned, early assignments in which the goal is to observe how people behave when stuttering occurs can do a great deal to invalidate predictions that there will be unhelpful audience reactions. The ability to make more positive predictions, based on the evidence collected whilst carrying out assignments, will go a long way to reducing anxiety.

There are occasions, however, when negative listener behaviours are encountered, and the person who stutters will clearly need some sort of effective strategy in dealing with bullying, teasing or other inappropriate reactions to stuttering. The problem-solving activity illustrated in Figure 5.1 – what to do when someone 'takes the mickey' – is a real-life example from an intensive course. It shows that the group brought considerable maturity and humour to bear on the problem, with nobody suggesting the younger children's option of 'beating them up'!

The second example, set out in Figure 5.2, is another real-life one. One of the older adolescent girls in the group was so scared and embarrassed about stuttering in shops that she would get her sister to shop for her. During one intensive course she admitted to needing a new pair of shoes and proposed asking her sister to accompany her and speak for her. We decided this was a good problem-solving topic, and it provoked some humorous, imaginative and illegal options for dealing with the situation. She was told that she could choose amd try out any alternative option (bar one). Interestingly, she selected and carried out the one which required most courage: she bought her own shoes!

Communication Skills

Many adolescents, through lack of social experience and lack of confidence, have poor social skills which will prevent them communicating effectively. This may occur only in more demanding and formal speaking situations, such as speaking in front of the class. We have found considerable variation in the social skills of adolescents who stutter, some appearing competent and confident and others greatly handicapped by their inability to deal with speech situations. Their abilities will tend to improve as the stutter reduces in severity, but we have found that placing considerable emphasis on these skills is an important and effective part of therapy.

The person who stutters, along with the majority of normal speakers, has probably not given very much thought to what is normal speech, or what constitutes effective speech. As Fransella (1972) observed, the stutterer has little in the way of constructs about normal speech, but a great

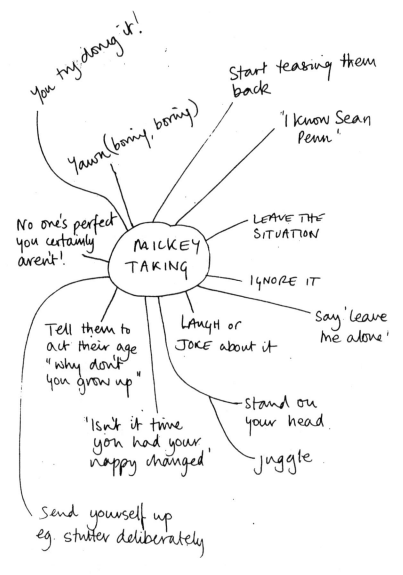

You try doing it!

Start teasing them back

Yawn (boring, boring)

'I know Sean Penn'.

No one's perfect you certainly aren't!.

MICKEY TAKING

LEAVE THE SITUATION

IGNORE IT

Tell them to act their age "why don't you grow up"

LAUGH or JOKE about it

Say 'leave me alone'

'Isn't it time you had your nappy changed'

Stand on your head.

Juggle.

Send yourself up eg. stutter deliberately

Figure 5.1 Problem solving 1: How to deal with teasing

many about stuttering. We therefore need to make him more aware of his own fluency and the positive aspects of his communication.

There are a number of ways in which this can be tackled. In the group situation this can be done with a 'brainstorming' session, posing questions such as 'What is normal speech?' or 'What makes a person communicate effectively?'. It is inevitable that the word fluency is mentioned, but the person who stutters is often unaware that there are other aspects of speech which can be equally important, such as intonation, facial expression and eye-contact. A demonstration by the therapist of the

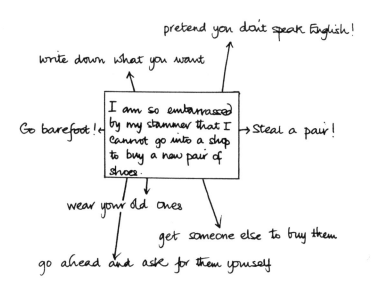

Figure 5.2 Problem solving 2: Some solutions to a dilemma

effect of poor communication skills on normal speech (by using a monotonous voice, looking away all the time and taking up a fixed posture) can be convincing evidence that fluent speakers are not necessarily good speakers. It can also be shown, with considerable effect, that even a person with a moderately severe stutter can be a very effective communicator. Some of the adolescents and adults in our groups have been surprised by their ability to give an interesting and amusing presentation in front of a group even though they were still stuttering. This is very important in improving self-esteem, and positive feedback from the peer group can be a powerful reinforcer in tackling more demanding situations.

In this way, we begin to highlight the normality of much of our clients' communicative behaviour. We are certainly beginning to shift the emphasis from stuttering to normal speech, so that the person who stutters can begin to build up some constructs of 'me as a normal speaker' and even of 'me as a good speaker'. All this will have considerable implications as he begins to tackle situations he has previously dreaded and avoided.

Assignments provide a very useful way of trying out improved communication skills, such as maintaining appropriate eye-contact. We can also make use of role play and informal and formal presentations in group therapy. Group members can give feedback on audibility, expressive use of voice, appropriate gesture and facial expression, as well as eye-contact. Most people who stutter have interesting things to say and worthwhile opinions to express, and the group may offer an opportunity to express what they really want to say for the first time. Speaking in front of a group (as in the classroom) is often regarded as a feared situation, and although we cannot simulate a large class in a small group, we can give experience of successful communication in front of an 'audience'. In fact, on the final afternoon of the intensive courses at City University, our group members perform in front of a classroom-sized audience of parents and other group members. The older members may give a presentation or be asked to comment on any gains they have made from the course. They may choose to read aloud in a situation previously avoided. Role plays, often centred on stuttering in some way, are performed; the role of the wicked teacher is a popular one, and unhelpful and impatient shop assistants, barmaids and booking office clerks provide material for entertaining parents! We consider that 'sending up' stuttering, whether in terms of adverse audience reactions or in terms of witty responses to bullying, are a very healthy development and are particularly indicative of changing attitudes when the ideas come from the group members themselves.

Fun as these activities are, for both performers and audience, they nevertheless provide some important issues for discussion after the performance is over. In particular, we need to impress on parents that having the confidence and the courage to 'perform' is far more important than some false and fragile fluency. Surprisingly or not, of course, the performers are often more fluent than they had predicted.

Increasing Linguistic Experiences

We have already mentioned Rustin and Klein's (1991) findings on the sometimes depressed linguistic competence of the adolescent who stutters. Whatever the reasons for this, we should take this into account in planning therapy. To some extent we are dealing with these problems in improving communication skills, but we can also help by increasing the adolescents' linguistic experience. This is, of course, achieved by carrying out assignments, particularly the more demanding ones of performing surveys and making extended telephone calls. Role-play activities can also achieve the same goal of improving linguistic competence. We also arrange for adolescent clients to interview and be interviewed, which is useful if they are seeking entry to further education or looking for a job.

Many of the adolescents' linguistic problems stem from lack of a variety of experiences, rather than a true deficit. In this way they are not very different from adolescents in general.

Measuring Progress

Most therapists involved in working with people who stutter have gone through the stage of feeling it is very important to do block counts and to time speaking or reading aloud. These do, of course, provide a very useful baseline for research, but are of limited value if one's goals are changing attitudes and achieving a more comfortable stutter. Block counting is a time consuming and artificial exercise when there are more important issues at stake.

How, then, can we measure and attempt to quantify progress? To some extent it depends on whom you want to impress! It is natural that parents, and indeed the client himself, want to see tangible evidence of progress, and there is nothing wrong with that. Therapists also need to be reassured that progress is being made, so that they can be confident in the efficacy of their methods.

We have found that the Perceptions of Stuttering Inventory (Woolf, 1967) is a fairly sensitive and reliable instrument, measuring levels of struggle, avoidance and expectancy, and most adolescents find it easy to complete the 60 items of the questionnaire. The results of each individual's struggle, avoidance and expectancy scores promote good group discussion and help to focus attention on goals to be achieved.

A fairly detailed profile of the individual's stutter is one of the more objective methods, against which future profiles can be compared. It should include both verbal and non-verbal behaviours which interfere with the speech process or merely add to the abnormality of speech. We can see a reduction in abnormal speech and non-verbal behaviours by comparing profiles made at the beginning and end of a course, or over two or more courses.

It is harder to quantify a reduction in avoidance, and yet this is probably one of the most important and sensitive indices of genuine improvement. The avoidance schedule given in the appendix at the end of this chapter can be used to give a clear idea of the client's pattern of avoidance, and is also useful in planning assignments.

One of the most subjective but revealing signs of progress is in the verbatim statements made by the client himself. A socially skilled and apparently 'laid back' adolescent recently described phoning as a 'nightmare' which gave a vivid impression of how he viewed that situation, with which any future comments could be compared. Subjective as such statements are, they represent the client's feelings on the subject and therefore have an intrinsic value which no amount of block counting can match.

As an intensive course progresses, we can see the increasing enthusiasm with which assignments are tackled. This is often mirrored by an increasingly creative approach to assignment planning, in which the group members are taking over the initiative from the therapists. We had a small sub-group of adolescents on a course who decided to plan a weekend for a party of American tourists. This included telephone enquiries to hotels and theatres, and even a visit to St Paul's Cathedral to find out the times of services, so that even the visitors' spiritual needs were met! This kind of activity tells us a good deal about the changes that are taking place in the growth of confidence and reduction of avoidance, but they are difficult to quantify. If we are to obtain a complete record of progress, however, these are important developments to note.

Parents may also provide very useful insights through their often unsolicited comments, and these may range from a new willingness to answer the phone to improved achievement at school. Sometimes it is a more global comment like 'He's a different boy'. Music, indeed, to any therapist's ears, but none the less such remarks may tell you as much about change of attitude in the parent and they are therefore worth noting.

To sum up on this difficult and indeed controversial area of stuttering, I will indulge in an expression of my own feelings, which are based on many years of practice in using both fluency-shaping and stutter-more-easily approaches. I am happier to see a young client – indeed, any client – confident in his or her ability to communicate effectively in spite of a stammer, than to see him or her go off on a high of fluency, with speech fears and avoidance unaddressed, and little idea of how to cope with failure when it happens, as inevitably it must. Attitude changes are far less susceptible to regression (Lawson *et al.*, 1993). It is not that one is ignoring fluency, or its importance to the client himself, but rather it is a realistic appraisal of the need to modify negative feelings about stuttering to underpin work on improving speech itself. Working in parallel to achieve a more comfortable stutter, for both the speaker and his audience, and to produce more positive attitudes about communication, has the compound effect of improving both, and we often see that the impetus of that change continues after the course has finished.

Progress is sometimes made in unexpected and exciting ways, as the following case studies show. This is not the stuff of which research is made, but is evidence of positive and important changes in the clients.

D.E. was 14 years old when he first came on a course. He was very sensitive about his stutter and went to considerable lengths to avoid using the telephone. The fact that he carried out a survey on stuttering for his GCSE, and presented his findings in front of his class, represented a tremendous achievement for D.E. The survey and some of the results are shown at the end of this chapter.

S.P. was a 17-year-old schoolgirl. She had a slight overt stutter, which caused her great embarrassment and distress. She attended courses and decided that she would probably train to be a speech therapist when she had completed her Psychology degree. At university she became involved with student Helpline and a drama group. She carried out her research project on stuttering. She graduated and decided to go into nursing, which was probably a braver move than speech therapy!

M.H. was 15 years old and attended two courses. She was very quiet and shy when she first came. Shortly after attending her second course she joined the Association for Stammerers as a volunteer in their office.

D.M., now 17 years old, attended two courses as a very diffident adolescent. Since then, he has chaired a discussion group of parents and their children who stutter, and has made himself available to come and talk to children attending intensive courses.

To meet the more stringent needs of research, perhaps we still need to count moments of stuttering in a variety of situations, and time output in speaking and reading. Riley's Stuttering Severity Instrument (1972) provides a standardised procedure for giving a subjective and more comprehensive overview of stuttering behaviour which can be used for measuring progress.

There is an urgent need for straightforward but sensitive question-naires which can be completed by clients, parents and teachers to assess progress in terms of attitudes and speech behaviours. These would certainly provide useful information which is currently largely ignored in efficacy studies.

Postscript

This chapter has elaborated on approaches and activities which may be employed in working with adolescents who stutter, preferably in a group setting. Much of what has been written will, however, apply in working with younger children and adults as the underlying philosophy holds good for all client groups.

References

Blyth, D.A., Simmons, R.G. and Carlton-Ford, S. (1983). The adjustment of early adolescents to school transitions. *Journal of Early Adolescence* 3(1–2), 105–120.

Brennan, T. (1982). Loneliness at adolescence. In: L. Peplau, and D. Perlman (Eds), *Loneliness: A Source of Current Theory, Research and Therapy*. New York: Wiley.

Brooks-Gunn, J. and Paikoff, R.L. (1992).Changes in self-feelings during the transition towards adolescence. In: H. McGurk (Ed.), *Childhood Social Development – Contemporary Perspectives*. Hillside, NJ: Lawrence Erlbaum.

Coleman, J.C. (1993). Understanding adolescence today: a review. *Children and Society* 7(2), 137–147.

Coleman, J.C.and Hendry, L. (1990). *The Nature of Adolescence*. London: Routledge.

Damon, W. (1983). *Social and Personality Development: Infancy through Adolescence*. New York: Norton.

Fransella, F. (1972). *Personal Change and Reconstruction*. London: Academic Press.

Hartup, W.W. (1982). Peer relations. In: C.B. Kopp and J.B. Krakow (Eds), *The Child: Development in a Social Context*. Reading MA: Addison Wesley.

Jackson, S. and Bosma, H.A. (1992). Developmental research on adolescence: European perspectives for the 1990s and beyond. *British Journal of Developmental Psychology* 10, 319–337.

Lawson, R. (1992). Groups with adults who stutter. In M. Fawcus (Ed.), *Group*

Encounters in Speech and Language Therapy. Leicester: Far Communications.

Lawson, R., Pring, T. and Fawcus, M. (1993). The effects of short courses in modifying the attitudes of adult and adolescent stutterers to communication. *European Journal of Disorders of Communication* **28**(3), 299–308.

Newman, P.R. and Newman, B.M. (1976). Early adolescence and its conflict: group identity vs alienation. *Adolescence* **11**, 261–274.

Riley, G.D. (1972). A Stuttering Severity Instrument for children and adults. *Journal of Speech and Hearing Disorders* **37**, 314–322.

Rustin, L. and Klein, H. (1991). Language difficulties in adolescent stutterers. *Human Communication* **1**(1), 15–16.

Sheehan, J.G. (1975). Conflict theory and avoidance-reduction therapy. In: J. Eisenson (Ed.), *A Second Symposium*. New York: Harper & Row.

Schwartz, H.D. (1993). Adolescents who stutter. *Journal of Fluency Disorders* **18**, 289–302.

Woolf, G. (1967). Perceptions of stuttering inventory. *British Journal of Disorders of Communication* **2**(2), 158–171.

Appendix I

Avoidance Schedule

Date Name						
Put a cross in the appropriate box to show how much you avoid. Do you avoid any of the following situations, and how often?						
Situations	Never	Seldom	Occasionally	Often	Very often	Always
Making telephone calls						
Answering the telephone						
Speaking in shops (empty)						
Speaking in shops (full)						
Asking for bus fares						
Asking for rail fares						
Speaking to strangers						
Asking the way						
Speaking to adults						
Speaking to people of your own age						
Speaking to young children						
Speaking to parents' friends						
Reading aloud in class						
Asking questions in class						
Speaking to your teacher						
Speaking to other teachers						
Speaking in a group of people						
Answering questions in class						

Appendix II

STUTTERING QUESTIONNAIRE

Name

Age: 0–10 ☐ 11–20 ☐ 21–30 ☐ 31–40 ☐ 41–50 ☐ 51–60 ☐ 61–70 ☐ 70+ ☐
How would you feel if someone came up to you and started to stutter?

Embarrassed ☐ Amused ☐ Bewildered ☐ Sympathetic ☐ Don't know ☐

Other   Reaction:

Why?

What is a stutter?

Do you consider stuttering a disability? Yes ☐ No ☐ Don't know ☐

If 'yes' why?

Would stuttering influence your judgement when choosing friends?

Yes ☐ No ☐ Don't know ☐ If 'yes' why?

Where do you go if you can't see properly?   An optician

Where do you go if you have a stutter?

How do you think people should be made more aware of speech impedements?

Thank you

Results of questionnaire (50 people answered)

How would you feel if someone came up to you and started to stutter?

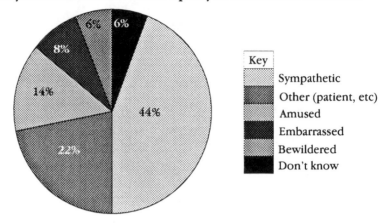

Do you consider stuttering a disability?

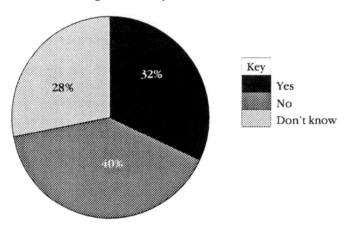

Would stuttering influence your judgement when choosing friends?

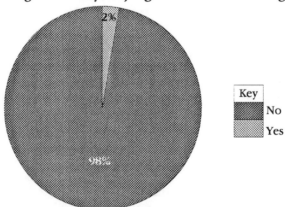

Pie chart to show age range of people surveyed

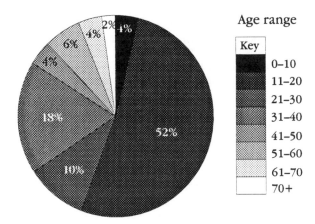

Age range

Key
- 0–10
- 11–20
- 21–30
- 31–40
- 41–50
- 51–60
- 61–70
- 70+

Bar graph to show expected reactions of people when they are approached by someone who sutters

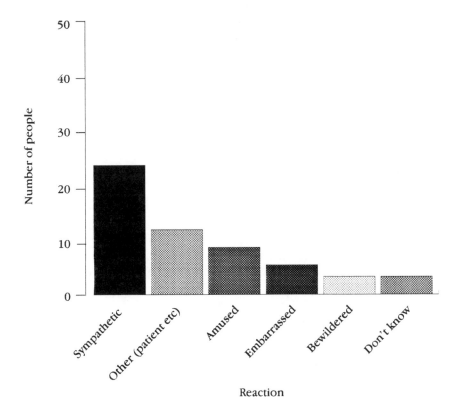

Basic assignment sheet 1

* Approach someone in the Department (Centre or School) to whom you have not already spoken. Introduce yourself, and find out their name and the work they are doing. Don't forget to thank them!

> Did you look at them when you spoke?
> Did you convey and obtain the information you wanted?
> How did you feel?

* Approach three people (one at a time) in the street. Ask them one basic question (e.g. 'What is the time?' 'Can you tell me where I can find the post-office?'). Remember to thank them!

> Did you feel the same in all three assignments?
> Did you get your qustion across?
> If you stammered, did people react in any way?

* Put the same basic question to six different people — three men and three women. Watch carefully how they react when you stammer.

> Did speaking to a man or a woman make any difference to you?
> What sort of reactions did you observe?
> What did you learn from this assignment?

Basic assignment sheet 2

* Go into a shop and make an enquiry. Ask at least two or three questions (e.g. in a baker's: 'How much are the doughnuts?' 'Do they have jam inside?'). Look at your listener and really listen to what he or she says. Thank him or her as you leave.

Do the same assignment in two other shops (or a museum, library or cinema).

> What did you learn from this?
> Did you feel different in each asignment?
> Were you more aware of your listener than usual?

* Make a phone call (to a hotel, for example) and ask one basic question (e.g. 'How much is a single room?'). Remember to thank the person at the other end when you finish.

> How did you feel when you had completed the assignment?
> Did you have to answer any questions?
> How did you feel before you picked up the phone?
> Did you suceed in asking your questions?

*Now make four more phone calls. Sit in a relaxed and comfortable position. Take your time when the person answers. Did you feel more in control of the situation?

Basic assignment sheet 3

* Make a further five telephone calls. This time, ask two or three questions. Remember your stategies for improving your performance (e.g. sitting in a relaxed way, not rushing to speak).

> Did you communicate successfully?
> Did you get thrown by any unexpected questions?
> How did you feel at the beginning and the end of this assignment?

*Try going into two situations where you stammer deliberately and obviously on two words. (e.g. 'Excuse me, can you tell me the time?').

> Did the listener react in any unusual way?
> How did you feel at the beginning and end of the assignment?

* Keep a record of your assignments, and what you observed and learnt from them. Remember to judge your performance on how well you communicated, and not on whether or not you stammered.

NOW PROCEED TO ADVANCED ASSIGNMENT SHEET 1.

Advanced assignment sheet 1

* Make a comparative study of your feelings in speaking to:

  a. Young people (e.g. children or teenagers)
  b. Older people (e.g. middle-aged or older)
  c. Men
  d. Women

* Try stammering quite deliberately and obviously with five different people, observing them as you do so.

> Did you feel in control of the situation?
> How did you feel before and after each assignment?
> What did you learn from this experience?

* Develop a natural conversation with someone. Imagine that you are encouraging them to talk. Ask them questions, listen carefully to the answers and develop the topic.

Has your awareness of the listener increased?
Did you feel in control of the situation?
What did you learn about yourself?

Advanced assignment sheet 2

*Decide on three situations where you can make a face-to-face extended enquiry. This could be in a travel agents, public library or railway station. Think through your first two or three questions, but try and ask one or two more that you have not prepared.

Were you successful in getting the information you wanted?
Did you really listen to the answers (and can you remember them!)?
How successfully did the other person communicate?

*Choose an area where you can obtain information on the telephone (e.g. about trains, theatre tickets or hiring a car). Plan — but don't rehearse your questions. Try and ask two or three questions on each phone call, and aim for ten phone calls.

Did your performance change as you went on?
Do you feel you are carrying out phone calls more competently?

*Choose a partner and plan a survey with them. Do not have more than three or four questions and make the survey as believable as possible. Aim to ask at least five people each, and make sure you both observe and evaluate each other's performance. Give feedback on each other's communication strengths and weaknesses.

Advanced assignment sheet 3

* Choose a different partner. Together plan an outing for a selected pair or group of people (e.g. a family, an American couple, a group of Japanese businessmen). Prepare the itinerary with all the relevant information (times and costs, etc). Start their programme about 9.30 a.m. and continue into an evening activity. You can use the phone as much as you like or go out and make the enquiries.

* Keep a record of your assignments. Rate your success as a communicator on an agreed scale (this will be discussed in your group). Be as objective as you can — carry out the assignments like an experiment which you are observing carefully. Think about the purpose of the assignments and what you have learned or gained from them.

Chapter 6
Group Therapy with Adults who Stutter

KHURSHEED BAJINA

Courage is doing what you're afraid of.

(Eddie Rickenbacker [1890–1973] Aviator)

The greatest mistake you can make in life is to be continually fearing you will make one.

(Elbert G. Hubbard [1856–1915])

When I started working with adults who stutter, I slipped every individual into the same basic programme of fluency-shaping techniques. As if they did not have enough problems, I converted them into monotonous, expressionless robots. I became more and more dissatisfied with my therapy, as the monotonous robots left my clinic only to become humans who stutterered as soon as they entered an anxiety-provoking situation. As I gained a working knowledge of personal construct psychology, and became familiar with Sheehan's iceberg and Van Riper's block modification techniques, I came to realise that fluency is only one issue in therapy. However, there is no doubt that most of my education came from discussion with the experts themselves, the people who lived their lives with a stutter. It became clear that feeling better about oneself and how one sees the world is a much firmer foundation on which to build fluency. Fluency-shaping techniques which do not address these covert issues are bound to create a structure that will collapse. Clients repeatedly reported feelings of failure when their techniques broke down, further destroying their self-esteem.

This chapter will attempt to give the working therapist a practical approach to running intensive stuttering groups, as well as introducing assertiveness training for people who stutter. The main goal is to get clients to move forward in their thinking, in their perception of their world and in their inter-personal communication. Desensitisation or fear reduction are important goals that can be achieved through experimentation. The clients who stutter will be called 'students' throughout the chapter, because they attended intensive courses as students.

99

A Theoretical Framework

The four stages of Van Riper's (1974) block modification therapy are used as a framework, with various therapy choices used at each stage. These include Kelly's (1955) personal construct therapy, and various other skills used for effective communication including assertiveness training. Self-esteem and other covert variables cannot be ignored in any course of therapy offered for people who stutter. Flexibility and catering to individual needs is the key to successful therapy, for 'by our frameworks we are hung' (Cooper, 1986).

Van Riper (1974) produced a programme which took the individual needs of the client into account and explored both the stuttering behaviour and the feelings or covert aspects and attitudes associated with stuttering. His block modification approach is composed of four stages: identification, desensitisation, variation and modification. In this chapter most of the tasks will refer to the first three stages, predominantly desensitisation and variation.

The Setting for Therapy

Our clients suffer a number of indignities throughout their lives so it is vitally important that we provide a setting where they are able to enhance their feelings of self-worth. The patient role in a health model automatically assumes that the professional is the expert and further reduces the patient to the role of the one in need of help or 'cure'. At City University, we have an educational setting where the expertise of the 'student' who has lived with the stutter is acknowledged.

Referrals are mainly received from speech and language therapists but self-referrals are also accepted and these often come through the Association for Stammerers. The intensive courses run at City University last for four or five days. The students are in the group to research their own subject of expertise with the guidance and facilitation of a professional therapist. The adult groups are varied in age, sex, socio-economic status and interests.

Experience has shown that the more varied the group the better it works. The 'gelling' or moulding of the group at the beginning of the course is a very important step in view of this variance. This first stage will be discussed further. A central common area where social communication can take place during breaks is an ideal setting for experimentation, which is a key feature in this therapy approach.

Therapy Tasks and their Rationale

In writing this chapter it had to be decided whether to write a totally task-orientated section preceded by a theoretical section, or to merge the two. It is important that our students know the rationale behind the tasks we ask them to perform. It was therefore decided to attach a theoretical rationale for each activity to the task itself, which makes it easier to substitute alternative tasks to achieve the same goals.

Group Introductions

It is important for the speech and language therapist to erase the student's perception that 'the therapist doesn't stutter so can't understand what we're going through'. We ask our clients to introduce themselves, knowing full well the difficulties of saying one's name. The first session is started with a word game (task 1). Each student is asked to think of a 'positive' adjective beginning with the same first letter as their name. This sets a positive tone and helps to remove the fear of initiating names, as well as introducing group members to one another.

In order to begin the gelling process, and to bring up issues of first impressions, group members are asked to look around the room and choose someone they would like to talk to. Most students admit that quite often they will 'know' if a person is going to be easy or difficult to talk to before they have even spoken to them. In their pairs, the students are asked to find out three things about each other and then introduce their partner to the whole group using the three pieces of information (task 2). The initial one-to-one interaction helps to desensitise the student when speaking to a stranger, but both have a common reason for being in the situation. Kelly (1970) cited in Hayhow and Levy (1989) viewed behaviour as our principal instrument of inquiry. In the group setting the students can give each other support in attempting interactions that are usually avoided. In a Kellyan sense we are encouraging the students to challenge their own predictions. The person who stutters is an 'expert' at hypothesising and predicting outcome without ever actually carrying out the experiment or basing his predictions on previous experiences. This usually brings a chuckle from the group as most of my students can relate to this phenomenon of the self-fulfilling prophesy without experimental research.

Group Expectations and Rules

In a group where there is such diversity, it is important for the members to voice behaviour that they find acceptable or unacceptable in a group setting, i.e. to come up with a set of group rules (task 3). The role of the therapist is to facilitate discussion and decision making and record the rules. Issues such as punctuality, interruptions, listening and verbosity, for example, are addressed. Negotiations should be encouraged during this task as this may be a new experience for students. Negotiating and entering a win–win situation is assertive behaviour and helps to raise self-esteem, which is another goal of therapy.

It is important for us as group facilitators to get a feel for the individual expectations of our group. Time is usually spent brainstorming hopes, fears and expectations (task 4). Plans for the week should not be carved in stone on day one of the course, and there should be sufficient flexibility to incorporate particular group needs. If the group has been moulded into a cohesive unit with these activities, then we have an excellent foundation on which to build the rest of the course.

The Block Modification Process

As stated before, stage one of the block modification process is identification. In this, stage one is identifying the stuttering behaviour. These are the features that are apparent to the eyes and ears of the listener. In order to set up a common vocabulary within the group we brainstorm all the possible behaviours such as blocks, repetitions, red face, tense shoulders, for example (task 5). Group members are then asked to pair up with a different partner, in order to expand their one-to-one experiences, and are asked to identify each other's stuttering behaviour and report what they observe to each other (task 6). There is then general discussion regarding how far the individual was aware of what the listener perceived, and any other issues arising from this task. There are often items that may be on the borderline between behaviour and feelings and these issues are also discussed.

Focusing on Communication

A brainstorm of 'What makes a good communicator?' (task 7) can follow. The topic is placed in a circle in the centre of the board and group members are invited to contribute their ideas. It is important that the therapist does not re-word these ideas, although a student may be asked to clarify their message on occasions. After the brainstorm is complete each item is considered in terms of whether it is a 'speech' or a 'non-speech' factor of communication. A number of students are so focused on 'speech' that this exercise often reveals that the non-speech aspects far outnumber the speech aspects in good communication.

Changing Perspectives

In the groups we are attempting to challenge the students' longstanding perspectives. This can be very threatening for them. When our major ways of making sense of the world in which we live are invalidated, we will feel threatened, because, if we accept the invalidation, we are going to have to engage in major reconstruction (Kelly, 1955, cited in Hayhow and Levy, 1989). If these invalidations are occurring in a sensitive and supportive setting, and in an active experimental way, it may reduce the anxiety, guilt and hostility and increase aggressiveness in a Kellyan sense. When we take the plunge and actively experiment and evaluate our construing, we are being aggressive (Kelly, 1955, cited in Hayhow and Levy, 1989). In other words we are encouraging our clients to 'go for it' rather than holding back.

Studying Speech

The group is encouraged to look carefully at fluent speech and the necessity to recognise the importance of what you say rather than how you say it. Using demonstration and diagrams the members of the group are introduced to the processes of phonation and articulation. They are encouraged to experiment in producing voiced and voiceless sounds and controlled blocks, gradually removing the mystery of sound production (task 8). Students have previously learnt or been told to use soft contacts, and these can now be encouraged in the context of in-block modification with the smooth release of the sound or words.

A session on diaphragmatic breathing is now included, not as a technique for fluency but as a relaxation tool and a means of increasing awareness of the mechanics of breathing and the control of expiratory air flow during speech. The blocking of this air flow is also demonstrated. This session can be followed by small-group work where the students can do more sound and word play with voiced and voiceless sounds as well as smooth release of 'difficult' sounds (task 9). As avoidance occurs at a sound, word and situational level it is important to experiment in all these areas.

Structuring Activities

It is important for each session to have a beginning and, more importantly, an end. The session should start with some active group game: 'Fruit Salad' is often a good choice (task 10).

The group chooses a topic (e.g. fruit or TV programmes) and each member of the group selects one name from that category. One student stands in the middle and that person's chair is removed. This student has to call out two of the items and the two named students have to change seats. As they are changing seats the centre student has to try to grab one of the available seats. If the centre student calls 'fruit salad' or TV Times' everyone has to change their seat.

This is a good desensitisation exercise where the student is put on the spot and has to think of two names quickly and call them out in front of a group, remembering where he or she is. It also starts the next session off on a positive and humorous note. Any party game can be adapted and used at the beginning of a session as long as it is fun, involves the whole group, and reduces fear of participating in a group interaction.

Assignments

It is important that a five-day course is not seen as beginning when the students arrive at the course location and ending when they leave each day. It is essential that the course should have continuity and that each day should end with a set of assignments.

On day one students might be asked to listen to the radio, watch TV or observe friends and family. They have to note down three good communicators and three bad communicators and why they have classed them as such. They are also asked to listen out for any disfluencies in so-called fluent or 'normal' speakers (task 11). It is valuable to have speech and language therapy student helpers in the group for small-group facilitation. The students are encouraged to set assignments for the facilitators in order that they may gain some experiential knowledge of stuttering.

On one particular course I was asked to walk up to a ticket collector at a station and stutter while asking for directions. I would recommend that therapists try this. My personal experience was quite devastating. I walked up to a collector at Euston station and asked him which train went to Apsley, with a massive block on Apsley. He went red and pointed to a train on a platform. I was totally flustered and unable to think straight so I just got on that train. It was not until the train started to move that I realised that I was on the wrong train. This stress is experienced by our students on a daily basis.

Setting the Scene for Change

The second day should also begin with a group cohesion exercise. Another fun name game is 'Spin the Plate' (task 12). All students and facilitators stand in a circle. One of the students has to spin the plate and call out someone else's name. The named person has to grab the plate before it stops spinning. This continues until everyone has had a turn.

To get an impression of the mood of the group, and to prepare the group for self-disclosure later in the day, each group member is asked to think of an animal that they feel like at that precise moment (task 13). They are asked to describe that animal and express how it is feeling. This will also provide a few individual constructs about members of the group.

If assignments have been set, feedback is the first item of the day. Each group member is encouraged to describe their observations and conclusions (task 14). This is a good time to discuss the various stages of carrying out an experiment, as well as the importance of acknowledging and sharing feelings. This activity will give the group a feeling of commonality as well as individuality. It will possibly change the two perspectives:

1. nobody else is like me and
2. you are either a fluent speaker or a 'stutterer' (there is a sharp dichotomy between the two groups).

Dealing with Feelings and Changing Perspectives

An important feature of the second day is the identification of feelings or the covert aspects of stuttering that the student experiences and of which the listener is often not aware. The group iceberg (task 15) is a very difficult as well as enlightening session for the students and some of the facilitators, as there is self-disclosure in a group of relative strangers. This is another reason why the gelling process is so important as there needs to be a sense of trust as well as camaraderie. Students are initially asked to brainstorm the covert feelings and the facilitator can write them in the iceberg 'under the surface of the water'.

Common words suggested are 'frustration... anger...anxious... feel stupid ... avoidance'.The facilitator writes down the student's words exactly as they are given. Students are then encouraged to relate experiences where they have felt the emotions listed under the iceberg. This is a good session for challenging and reframing perspectives. The facilitator may be able to offer alternative possibilities for the student's construction of or perspective on an event (task 16). The student tends to make a number of assumptions about the listener such as:

...he looked away because he thought I was stupid.

An alternative view offered could be that none of us is brought up knowing how to communicate with a person who stutters, and this person may have been anxious and confused and not sure of how to react. This is also a good time to discuss educating public opinion. The students often have unrealistic expectations of people who are in fact ignorant about the stuttering syndrome. For some students this is the most crucial session of the course.

Dealing with Avoidance

The group iceberg session is in its very nature desensitising as the students are confronting their fears and beginning reconstruction. Following on from earlier discussions about anticipation, avoidance and situational anxiety, there is more discussion around these terms in order to develop a common language as well as to challenge negative constructs. A firm group rule should be 'GO FOR IT'. No student is allowed to avoid a word if it is the one they really want to use. This is most difficult for the more covert students.

There is a strong correlation between anxiety and self-esteem (Bajina, 1992) and a factor that may contribute to this association is the tendency for people with low self-esteem to present a false front to the world. A number of the students have made a career of learning how to avoid words in order that they appear to be fluent speakers. Most of these students have forgotten how to be themselves. It is difficult to fix or modify something if you cannot see what needs to be fixed. It is fair to warn them that they will initially feel extremely uncomfortable as they are being asked to break down the wall of defences and coping strategies they have spent their whole lives building up.

One of the assignments for the evening may be to write down and rank 10 or 12 situations which cause the students anxiety. This can also be a productive group activity. As the aim of the course is to reduce fear through experience and experiment, it is useful to introduce role play of these feared and often avoided situations. This is an ideal way to set up anxiety-provoking situations to be faced in a relatively safe environment. Groups of three work well as each student can take a turn at being an observer and reporter while the other two carry out the role play.

Encouraging a more Objective Approach

Students often start by placing blame on the general public for not being good listeners or not being sensitive to their predicament. It is important for the students to start taking responsibility rather than attaching blame. If the blame is laid on someone else, or stuttering is seen as something that 'happens to me', then the student has given up control as well as the motivation to change things. If, however, the students learn to take control of their own lives by accepting responsibility and thinking of stuttering as something they do, then they can begin to change and move forward.

A task designed to promote more accurate observation could involve dividing into pairs or having two rows facing each other and partnering the person opposite (task 17). One student is the observer and the other is the actor. The actor is asked to stand in a particular way and the observer notes facial expression and body posture. The observer then turns away from the actor who is asked to change three things about their pose and/or expression. The observer then turns his back and has to detect the changes. Roles are then reversed. Students often jump to hasty conclusions or have a number of prejudices about their 'fluent' listeners without taking time to listen or really observe them. One of my favourite quotes 'prejudice saves a lot of time, because you can form an opinion without the facts', is often relevant to people who stutter and increases anticipation and avoidance.

Dealing with Negative Feelings within the Group

As the main facilitator, it is important that the therapist is aware of the mood of the group. With experience it is possible to pick up discomfort or things unsaid. This can produce a negative atmosphere and should be dealt with as soon as possible. A number of our students carry 'baggage' filled with anger and resentment and this may manifest itself in a number of ways. Any therapist working with adults who stutter should at least have basic counselling skills and a knowledge of group dynamics and facilitation.

C.T. was a very angry 26-year-old. She was a very covert stutterer who had become an expert at avoidance and was rarely able to say what she really meant or felt. After one lunch break we began our session and it was clear that she was seething. This was being picked up by the group and it had to be addressed. They were reminded of the rule about being open and expressing anything that was making them angry or uncomfortable.

C.T. stood up, pointed at a group member and said 'all right then, he's sitting in my seat'. This immediately defused the atmosphere and made for a more pleasant afternoon. We are all guilty of going on courses and keeping the same chair or space throughout. As human beings we all need some degree of familiarity and predictability.

Experimentation and Desensitisation

Assignments for days two to five are all experimentation and desensitisation tasks. They may be as varied as phoning directory enquiries or ordering a drink in a pub. All experimentation involves all four stages of the modification process. Identification is an ongoing process and in Kellyan terms reconstruction and elaboration of constructs is continuous throughout the stage of variation.

Making video recordings is an excellent way for students to observe their stuttering behaviour and how they appear to their listener. Video feedback has been used as early as the second day with a well-gelled group. Each student is asked to speak for three minutes on a topic which particularly interests them. This is often a good exercise for the end of the day so that feedback and discussion can be carried out the following morning (task 18).

The facilitator must make it clear that the first observations have to be reported by the student who has been filmed, after which other members may make constructive observations. The students are encouraged to make as many positive observations as negative ones. Group tasks on the giving and receiving of compliments arise naturally out of this activity (task 19).

Encouraging Awareness of Non-verbal Aspects of Speech

In order to move the focus from speech one can employ a task called 'In the manner of the word' (task 20). Each student is given an adverb or an emotive word such as 'angrily' or 'surreptitiously', written on a piece of paper so that the rest of the group cannot see it. The group gives the student with the paper an action such as digging or driving and the student does this in the manner of their word. A particularly hilarious session ensued when one of our more inhibited students had to drive 'passionately'. This is an excellent task after a particularly heavy session. There is a release through laughter and there is no obligation to speak in order to get your message across.

Trying out Speech and Predictions in the Group

No matter how much you want to steer your group away from speech, the reality is that when they leave the group that is their main mode of communication. Students have reported that they find the small-group work, where they can play with sounds and words, very useful. This is a further important part of desensitisation. Voluntary stuttering is often tried out in these small groups. The group may be provided with written material and engage in a task that attacks anticipation and the self-fulfilling prophesy. Students are asked to mark the words in a passage on which they expect to have difficulty. The new rule is that they are allowed to stutter voluntarily on the word after their chosen word. Again this task (task 21) challenges their belief that they can always predict when they are definitely going to have difficulties.

The students have already ranked their situation hierarchies and should be allowed to attempt their anxiety-provoking situations either through role play or using real-life situations.

Lawson (1992) describes the use of obstacle courses. One of the facilitators is blindfolded and guided through an obstacle course of tables and chairs set up by the students (task 22). The students are told that the blindfolded individual is a robot and needs small, specific directions, e.g. move your left foot two inches to the right. The robot will not respond to a message if there is any avoidance, back-tracking or the use of fillers. This task puts each student on the spot. They are not allowed to avoid and have to go for the exact words. They are told that the robot will respond to a word that has been released after a block as long as the student has attempted it. We are asking students to think and speak in a group situation where their message is important and has consequences. For many this would be very high on their list of feared situations but this fear is defused by the group goal and the fun of causing the facilitator as much grief as possible.

If you are in a setting such as City University it is possible to capture a lecturer to provide an opportunity for the students to carry out a mock interview with a stranger. This is done on day four or five when confidence is high. If there are other groups running at the same time some students may like to do presentations or just answer questions from other students or facilitators.

Educating the Public

During the course there is considerable discussion about prejudices and assumptions on the part of the person who stutters and members of the public. One of the final activities (task 23) on the course is the creation of a survey by the group to check out some of their assumptions about what the public think. The students go out in pairs and intercept members of the public. Feedback after this experiment is usually extremely positive and often the students have begun the process of education.

Negotiation and Confrontation

A final task (task 24) which involves negotiation, confrontation and good communication in a group setting is the 'Balloon Debate'. A number of occupations are written on pieces of paper, and one is handed to each student. It is more fun if there are some controversial choices such as a politician or a nun or a tightrope walker. All the people are in a hot air balloon that is leaking and is sinking fast. Only one person may remain in the balloon to live and tell the tale. All the others must jump out into the ocean so that the balloon can reach land safely. Each person has to make an argument for why they should remain in the balloon based on what they can do for mankind. There is an initial round of statements from each group member and then the interactions begin. Everyone suggests reasons for someone else to jump. At the end of the debate there is a vote as to who should stay in the balloon based on the quality of their argument. This exercise involves all the social and communication skills learnt over the course of the week. Students have to initiate conversation, turn-take, and express their opinions. Group rules may have to be reiterated if discussion gets heated.

The Final Session

Lawson (1992) has commented that the final moments of a group are often full of an intense mixture of feelings, and it is important that there is some attempt at a debriefing session.

It is useful for students to look back at their original expectations and to see how far these have been achieved. It is important for the therapist to have feedback on how successful the group was for each student, as his or her therapy and group management can only benefit from honest feedback.

Ending on a positive note, each student is given the chance to pay each member a compliment. Lawson (1992) has suggested that the group makes a video, in which all take part and which is a 'lighthearted look at themselves and the course'.

The students are recommended to have follow-up therapy from their local therapist. They are encouraged to continue the process of the course by experimenting in different and more difficult situations and finally to 'GO FOR IT!'.

The timing of different tasks is offered as a guide for therapists who are new to running 'stutter-more-fluently' groups. Therapists will acquire their own style and plan and will discover new tasks as they gain experience.

References

Bajina, K. (1992). An investigation of the covert aspects associated with the 'Stuttering Syndrome' – a reinforcement model. Unpublished MSc thesis, City University, London.

Cooper, E.B. (1986). Joseph G. Sheehan's contributions: an eagle soars. *Journal of Fluency Disorders* 11, 175–182.

Hayhow, R. and Levy, C. (1989). *Working with Stuttering*. Oxford: Winslow Press

Kelly, G.A. (1955). *The Psychology of Personal Constructs*. New York: Norton.

Lawson, R. (1992) Groups with adults who stutter . In: Fawcus, M. (Ed.), *Group Encounters in Speech and Language Therapy*. London: Whurr Publishers.

Sheehan, V.M. (1986). Approach avoidance and anxiety reduction. In: Shames, G.H. and Rubin, H., *Stuttering Then and Now*. Seattle: Charles E. Merrill.

Van Riper, C. (1974). Modification of behaviour. In: Starkweather , C.W. (Ed.), *Therapy for Stutterers*, (pp. 45–61). Speech Foundation of America Publication No.10.

Chapter 7
Personal Construct Theory in Use with People who Stutter

ROBERTA WILLIAMS

In his description in 1955 of constructive alternativism, Kelly proposed that 'it is not a matter of indifference which of a set of alternative constructions one chooses to impose upon his world. Constructs cannot be tossed about willy-nilly without a person's getting into difficulty....The yardstick to use is the specific predictive efficiency of each alternative construct and the overall predictive efficiency of the system of which it would, if adopted, become a part.' In this chapter, stuttering will be examined as if it is a 'poor implement' of alternative construing and therapy will be reviewed as a method of reconstruction; a means of improving the overall predictive efficiency of the system.

Those who have become familiar with Personal Construct Theory (PCT) over the years will be aware of its enormous influence on speech and language therapists working with people who stutter. It has invited and permitted them to understand, almost, what it is like to stutter and to appreciate the implications for change for clients. From their work with PCT some therapists have moved into full-time counselling work whilst others remain as speech and language therapists with enhanced confidence and improved methods for working with different clients (not only people who stutter).

The very helpful relationship between PCT and stuttering first became known in 1970 with the publication of 'Stuttering: not a symptom, more a way of life' by Fay Fransella. This article encapsulated her research, later published in 1972, which examined the effect of increasing the meaningfulness of fluency for the person who stutters and was enriched by the detailed account of therapy with Luke. Since then, the role of PCT with people who stutter has been further elaborated by, amongst others, Dalton (1983) and Hayhow and Levy (1989) in their invaluable contributions. For many stuttering therapists, PCT provided a lifeline, because often the problem of stuttering did not seem to respond to behavioural techniques. As Hayhow and Levy (1989) noted, therapy seemed to be 'the roundabout of technique–practice–failure–

recrimination–more practice–failure and so on'. In addition, speech and language therapists were, in general, not adequately educated in methods to facilitate attitude change. PCT was and is important because it does not provide 'something to do' to the client but is a framework from which the therapist and the client can view the stuttering problem as it is, rather than how we are told it might be. It is a theory and, as Kelly states, 'a theory may be considered as a way of binding together a multitude of facts so that one may comprehend them all at once'. Stuttering seems to be a 'different' problem for each client and therefore presents constantly new data for the therapist, some of which fit the stereotype and more that do not! PCT is appealing because it is a person-centred approach which illuminates the very personal ways in which stuttering is experienced. It is not a technique to be applied, but instead provides a structure for the experimenters, both client and therapist, through which they can try out different behaviours and evaluate their 'fit' or implications.

In that a certain degree of knowledge is assumed in the reader, the theory itself will be described only briefly within this chapter, highlighting the main areas of attention. Greater explanation and detail is richly provided in such texts as those by Dalton and Dunnet (1989), Winter (1992), Hayhow and Levy (1989) and, of course, Kelly (1955). The bulk of this chapter will look at the phenomenon and treatment of stuttering in people of all ages through the framework of personal construct theory, although the focus will lean towards working with adults. This is because the understanding of a child is subsumed under the understanding of people. Naturally, techniques for eliciting constructs from young children are different from those used with adults but principles of therapy through the use of the PCT framework remain the same.

Personal Construct Theory

Most importantly, Kelly's theory was about people and about change. The relevance of the theory is not limited to the clients or 'subjects' but includes the professionals employing the theory. Each person is seen as a scientist in his or her own right conducting their own experiments and each person takes responsibility for how change can come about. They are not just the victims of chance stimuli. Although constructive alternativism stated that change is always potentially possible, Kelly described in great detail why changes may not be made or why they may be difficult. People are recognised as complex beings with intricate construct systems. The term construct is used as the most fundamental unit within the structure and is the device through which discriminations are made. A construct can be concrete or abstract, exists at different levels of awareness and is as important for its position within the person's construct system as for its content. Kelly's fundamental postulate and eleven corollaries describe the content and structure of the construct system, stressing all the time the importance of constant movement and change. This change is further elaborated in three cycles. First we **learn**, which Kelly described in the **experience** cycle and which involves, essentially, the organised testing out of constructs in the face of an event for validation or invalidation. If the expected outcome is disconfirmed there is constructive revision. The second cycle is **creativity** which is the process of moving constantly from loose to tight to loose construing and the third is the **CPC** cycle. This concerns decision making where the person starts with circumspection, moves through pre-emption and ends with control.

Using PCT with people who stutter, as with anyone, necessitates understanding the person in their own terms, i.e. subsuming their construct systems, and this is where the theory or 'framework for understanding problems and possibilities' (Fransella and Dalton, 1990) is so valuable. Kelly states that we are looking for 'bridges between the client's present and his future' and calls this process the transitive diagnosis. To do this, a therapist suspends his or her own value system and adopts the credulous approach, attempting to construe through the client's structure, with the help of professional constructs. Professional constructs are the keystone to diagnosis and therapy, the framework through which to investigate where someone may be employing inefficient construing and through which to design and plan for reconstruction. In other words the therapist tries to gain better understanding of the client and evolve jointly planned changes.

Using Professional Constructs to Make a Transitive Diagnosis

It is informative to observe the level of cognitive awareness at which someone is construing. Constructs which are at a high level are readily expressed; both alternatives are accessible and fall within the range of convenience of the client's major constructions. However, the fluent pole of the construct 'stuttering–fluent' is sometimes not readily accessible or is submerged for the stuttering person, meaning that elaboration of this pole is difficult or inadequately achieved. A client may see all fluent people as, for example, 'ambitious', 'successful' and 'unrestricted', but very little else – they do not seem to be real people at all. The pole of fluency is certainly not construed in a propositional fashion. By noting how lopsided a person's system is, it can be understood better by the therapist why the individual maintains the known but undesirable symptom.

Professional construing involves analysing the type of constructs used, noting what is core or central for the person and what is peripheral, and whether constructs are permeable or not to new events. Observing the use of **pre-emptive**, **constellatory** or **propositional** constructs again allows the therapist access to why changes may not be made. For example, if someone who stutters sees fluent people pre-emptively as *nothing but* 'good speakers' and otherwise 'shallow', it may explain why they are resistant to change in this direction.

Sometimes clients find it hard to articulate their feelings or they behave in a way which is inconsistent with their goals. This may indicate that a level of **pre-verbal construing** is being employed, often related to dependency issues from the past and which keeps an individual from making changes.

Noting the presence or absence of **dilation** or **constriction**, **loose or tight construing** or whether someone is stuck in any part of the **cycles of change** as mentioned previously are all uses of the framework through which we subsume the client's system. In addition, Kelly suggests we observe how the promise of change affects us through his description of further **dimensions of transition**. These include:

- **anxiety:** awareness that events are outside the range of convenience of the construct system, i.e. they cannot be construed by the system as it stands;
- **threat:** the awareness of an imminent comprehensive change in one's core constructs. For example Fransella's client, Luke, experienced threat in therapy because there were insufficient implications for being without his speech problem;
- **guilt:** the awareness of dislodgement of self from one's core role structure. A very powerful diagnostic construct, this explains resistance to 'instant' fluency. It feels odd and dislodges the person from everything that they know best;
- **fear:** the awareness of an imminent incidental change in one's core structures;
- **aggression:** the active elaboration of one's perceptual field;
- **hostility:** the continued effort to extort validational evidence in favour of a type of social prediction which has already been recognised as a failure.

To conclude, by **suspending** or putting 'on hold' the therapist's own construct system, he or she is freed to examine credulously the other person's construct system through the use of professional construct support. Fransella and Dalton (1990) is recommended for further reading in this area and, in a later section in this chapter, the characteristics of stuttering will be examined using this framework.

PCT and Personal Growth and Change in the Speech and Language Therapist – in Education and Afterwards

By providing an abstract framework, the metatheory of PCT offers something akin to grid references and symbols on a map whereby alternative ways through or round unexpected terrain can be plotted by therapist and client working together. For the speech and language therapist not trained in psychotherapy or advanced counselling skills, having the confidence to examine someone else's map and understand this person in their own terms is vital if any proposed changes are to be meaningful for them. Although these abstract guidelines are particularly useful for understanding the processes operating in therapy they also provide a reference for the therapist's own reactions because of the reflexive nature of the theory. Student speech and language therapists obtain an education in both the description of speech and language disorders, including stuttering, and the flexible way in which therapy is approached. However, it would seem that even greater attention could be paid, beneficially, to the principle of transitive diagnosis, especially with stuttering. A large number of speech and language therapists confess they are anxious about taking on people who stutter. Reasons are many and varied but often include an awareness on the part of the therapist that events are outside the range of convenience of their own system. One suspects that this is because, as mentioned before, people who stutter are so dissimilar and rely on very different therapeutic approaches in order to facilitate change. What is more, some may and do feel that it is not actually a problem at all. In other words, a good knowledge of the disorder *per se* is not necessarily enough: one needs a strong background in appreciating the numerous ways in which the 'disorder' is perceived by each person. PCT can provide a useful and manageable framework for the new therapist in dealing with the notion of variety within client groups and appeals to 'common sense' that people do not respond similarly to the same therapy.

From a broader perspective, the student speech and language therapist must often undertake quite comprehensive construct system revisions, for example when first handling people in distress or when first confronting permanent physical or mental change in various different client groups. The dimensions of transition are never more obvious than in the change taking place during active learning, and the promotion of insight into growth and development is one of the most powerful parts of education of any form. Students and qualified therapists are continually subject to revisions of their professional construct systems as they face the challenges of their work. Transition is part and parcel of education. Just as clients need support through the process of change, so therapists also need an opportunity to reflect on revisions to their personal construct systems if they are to continue to grow and develop professionally.

PCT and Stuttering

The next section will examine the nature of disorders, stuttering in particular, and suggest ways of understanding some of the difficulties and blocks to change that exist for the person who stutters. Some phenomena, seen as common to all stuttering, will be discussed in PCT terms in order to observe the alternative constructions which might be placed upon the reasons for their existence.

What is a Disorder?

Kelly (1955) said that a disorder could be called 'any personal construction which is used repeatedly in spite of consistent invalidation'. In a summary of his chapter on structural disorders, Winter (1992) expands on this, stating that the disorder's 'symptoms may represent aspects of the experience of invalidation, such as the anxiety or state of arousal associated with an inability to predict events; or manifestations of the persistent and exclusive use of a particular strategy in an attempt to cope with invalidation. The various contrasting strategies which the individual may employ for this latter purpose form the basis for a taxonomy of structural disorders of construing.'

Is Stuttering a Disorder?

Some individuals who stutter do not regard it as a 'disorder' and do not seek therapy. They accept it, presumably as something they do that is slightly outside the norm for their culture but which has not had implications for the other parts of their lives. Stuttering is, however, definitely seen as a 'different' way of speaking by many people, both fluent and disfluent, but it is important that a therapist should bear the possible acceptability of stuttering in mind and allow clients to set their own boundaries.

The decision about whether stuttering is a disorder sometimes depends on the apparent severity of the problem although this has its own drawbacks as a guideline. For example, it may seem to other people, including the family and the therapist, that the stuttering is not overtly severe whilst to the person concerned it is really disabling. Here it is vital that the person's construction of their problem is attended to rather than the symptom's face value alone.

Winter (1992) describes 'disorders' from two angles. Either individuals are seen as elaborating their systems in the problem area or, because their systems are elaborated in this area, they are expressing distress through a symptom which is consistent with these constructions. In the description of stuttering, Fransella (1972) tends to favour the latter and draws upon the choice corollary to explain stuttering. This states that 'a person chooses for himself that alternative in a dichotomised construct through which he anticipates the greater possibility for extension and definition of his system'. In other words 'a person stutters because he knows how to do it'. Stuttering is the behaviour that has received the most attention over the years and it has a finely tuned organisation of constructs. Its fatal flaw is that it is unreliable as a predictive tool. Constructs related to stuttering are increasingly tightened up or 'battened down' to prevent leakage or unreliability until the whole construct system is centred on the unwelcome behaviour. When the symptom starts to take over to any degree it is usually perceived as a problem by the individual concerned.

Therefore, whether stuttering is or is not labelled a 'disorder' may indeed be a matter for the person who does it. If, using Kelly's terminology, a person regards her 'stuttering self' as being at odds with her core constructs about herself, i.e. with guilt, then she may indeed be viewed as using a personal construction repeatedly despite consistent invalidation – that is, as having a disorder. If, however, constructs about stuttering fit with the whole person just as something they do rather than invalidating or dominating their core constructs then the phenomenon need not be perceived with the accompanying 'disorder' label.

Explanation of Some Stuttering Phenomena in PCT Terms

Why Stutter?

The search for the origins of stuttering in any individual has been under way probably since the first person perceived themselves as 'stuttering'. 'Causes' have been sought in the areas of learning theory and psychogenic and organic disorders but, as yet, there is no firm proof to commit us to any one line. Fransella (1972) used personal construct theory to explain that, in the beginning, stuttering develops because the child, observant of his own and others' reactions to his awkward early attempts to talk, learns to discriminate between disfluency and fluency and slowly elaborates his constructions of disfluency more than the constructions of fluency. As the child perceives that both internal and external responses to the act of stuttering are negative so he or she tries to stop. This act of stopping, however, involves effort and disruption of the automatic sequence and increases tension. Rather than reducing stuttering it actually increases it. In spite of this, the individual may have learned, in a variety of ways, to understand him- or herself best from the vantage point of those poles which best describe them as someone who stutters. For example, a person may feel he or she is a 'good listener', 'sensitive' and even 'academic'. If they are forced to concentrate on stuttering in an effort to control and predict it to such a degree that their system becomes constricted and tightened then gradually the view of the world may be construed from the viewpoint of stuttering alone and the 'overall predictive efficiency', of which the alternative construct 'stuttering' is part, may certainly not produce optimum functioning in the person.

If the system is really polarised, it may be that any experiment with adopting fluency would carry with it the baggage of 'unpredictable' and 'uncontrolled' or even 'poor listener', 'insensitive' and 'non-academic' and we can see how approaching life through the 'problem' probably influences growth and variation of construing in other areas. For example, a young woman recently receiving therapy for stuttering was in a dilemma about how to construe her new boyfriend's stuttering. She herself was working on reconstruing what it is like to be a fluent person and she realised she was feeling more and more critical of his stuttering. It appeared, after some discussion, that the old meaning of 'fluent person' implied 'critical of stuttering', an implication which needed revising, first, to make 'being a fluent person' an attractive choice for her and, second, to prevent a breakdown in her relationship! Through this discussion, new insight was gained into the power of tightly held constellatory constructs. In a hostile way she was supporting her view that it is better to stutter and be nice than to be fluent and critical of stuttering and once this implicative dilemma was raised to an appropriate level of awareness something could be done to effect change.

Why be Fluent?

In order to understand the development of stuttering, we need to address the way in which PCT looks at the development of fluency. It is assumed that a baby first discriminates elements in its environment without labels and that during the first and second years of life phonological and grammatical structures are organised and attached to these discriminations. Initial attempts at speech are almost invariably erroneous and are often found amusing and charming by those close to the developing child. They are certainly paid attention to, corrections are made by adults and older children, sometimes quite strictly, and in normal development the acceptable targets are gained. Why then does attention paid to abnormal forms by a carer not lead to maintenance of this behaviour as we are told it does to stuttering or, conversely, why does the presence of some fluency not lead to more fluency in the stuttering child? To continue the argument from the previous section, it may be that disruptions of prosody and behaviours that are stammer-like seem 'wrong' or 'disordered' and provoke tension in the speaker and the listener. It may be this tension which is elaborated and attended to most fully, creating unpredictable anticipation. We cannot, however, label tension firmly as the root cause because there is no evidence to support this. There is some evidence to support an organic or constitutional basis for stuttering (see Curlee and Perkins, 1985 for a review) and it may be that, as Van Riper (1982) feels, the various stresses placed upon an already fragile mechanism can tip the balance into stuttering. As usual there are no ready answers to these questions but it is vital that the nature of fluency is not left out of the equation. Starkweather (1987) defines fluent speech along the parameters of continuity, effort, rate and rhythm and it may be that while any one of these is not disrupted too extremely then neither is the speaker nor the listener. Once the disruption becomes too great, tension may be added to the mixture and speech is perceived as abnormal. The listener must always be included in the equation because, without him or her, again there would be no problem.

It is always astonishing how far the range of acceptable disfluency extends and we assume that, in general, people have construct systems which accommodate simple speech errors and can discriminate quite easily between slips of the tongue, normal hesitations and stuttering. Invariably the listener and the person stuttering can always tell if errors are exceeding their boundaries. On questioning it always seems that the 'extremeness' of the speech error is not the only factor: it must be accompanied by a *feeling*, for example, of tension or of being 'out of control'. Leitner (1981) describes the way in which every construct has a feeling, a behavioural and a value component so that, in the case of disfluency, the 'stuttering' is the (external) behaviour, 'out-of-control' is the (internal) feeling and 'not acceptable' may be the (internal and external) value. Prins (1993) also outlines the ways in which theorists from widely different backgrounds have conceived of stuttering events as comprising two main components. First there are 'covertly perceived interruptions of speech fluency signalled by cues associated with speech production and experienced by stutterers as a loss of control' and, second, there are 'coping defence reactions' to these cues (the stuttering behaviours). He stresses that, unless a person has a conviction that their skills are adequate the signal cues will continue to arouse powerful defence reactions. According to Prins, our treatment emphasis should therefore, be on the person's level of conviction rather than on the level of skill he possesses.

Stuttering Problems viewed through the PCT Framework

People who stutter may be experiencing problems with:

(a) the content of their constructs;
(b) the structure of their construct system; or
(c) both.

In other words, their lives may be affected by the use of limited and impermeable discrimination about some things and/or the way the rest of their experiences and constructs are organised and bound to the constructs of stuttering. It is important to reiterate that, in some people, stuttering does not greatly affect them and it is not perceived as a disorder. The following list, whilst by no means exhaustive, briefly sketches some of the findings from individuals who do present for therapy:

1. People who stutter seem to have two views of themselves – unlike other stutterers when not speaking, but like others who stutter when speaking (Fransella, 1972).
2. People who stutter tend to construe tightly rather than loosely. An individual, for example, might see success at work, sense of self-worth, ability to join social sports clubs, attractiveness to the opposite sex, loyalty and sensitivity all from the stuttering viewpoint in spite of their apparently divergent content. This may relate to Sheehan's (1970) 'giant in chains' theory which states that some people who stutter view stuttering as the only reason they are held back from success in all areas. Tight construing may be the only way someone feels they can keep in control but it is also likely to prevent change. Because stuttering is so unpredictable, the person may tighten their system increasingly in order to gain control over it.
3. People who stutter may tend to use pre-emptive and constellatory constructs rather that propositional constructs about stuttering. They may feel they can only predict events in terms of 'being a stutterer' or reacting as a stuttering person. Stuttering, however, may carry with it the predictions of embarrassment, awkwardness and avoidance, reactions which often occur with little variation. According to Kelly, without variation there is no experience, no learning and no chance of change.
4. As previously described, the pole of 'fluency' may be submerged or poorly elaborated: meaningless. If the direction of change has no solid foundation, then, however attractive it may be, it will be too difficult to approach.
5. Anxiety (the awareness that events are outside the range of convenience of the system) is a common experience for people who stutter and may be due to the unpredictability of the disfluency. When about to enter a speaking situation, people may be uncertain about whether they will or will not stutter as well as how this may be manifest. He or she may have tried to control all possible scenarios so that the likelihood of disfluency is reduced but there is often great stress about whether something unexpected will interfere. If this does happen or if anticipation and effort leads to extreme tension, the person's system may be so tight that the only alternative to controlled fluency is uncontrolled stuttering. What is interesting is that then anxiety can be reduced because the prediction of stuttering has been validated and the actual manifestation established. This theory supports Shee-

han's (1970) Fear Reduction Hypothesis which states that this reduction of intense emotion following blocking behaviour actually contributes to the reinforcement of the behaviour. The fact, however, that stuttering produces unpredictable listener reactions continues the process of anxiety. Anxiety is, unfortunately, not limited to the stuttering behaviour, but also influences the person's interpretation of fluency, an important point if we are to address why fluent speech does not invalidate stuttering. Without sufficient elaboration of the implications that fluency has for the person, everything about it lies outside the range of convenience for the individual and no firm predictions can be hypothesised. Therapists will recognise the profound disappointment experienced when, thrilled with the fluent performance of one of their clients under difficult circumstances, they find that the client himself does not feel it was real or has put it down to luck. The constant switching between ability and inability to predict events would appear to contribute to the state of constant anxiety complained of by people who stutter. Hayhow and Levy (1989) note that, 'people who stutter have a need for certainty and predictability. Because speaking is one of the most important ways of presenting ourselves, it is understandable that people who stutter become focused on speech and translate all their uncertainties into anxiety about stuttering.' This may mean, of course, that concentration on the minutiae of speech can divert from the wider issues about a conversation, for example how they are perceived as a whole, which the person who stutters may feel are too anxiety producing.

6. It may be that Kellyan hostility is operating in the above scenario where the client feels that the fluency was 'lucky'. Even when fluent, the person will probably be trying to gain evidence to support stuttering predictions and will 'cook the books' in order to preserve control.

7. In addition to anxiety, it is not uncommon for the individual also to feel threatened by any new fluency. Core constructs are being challenged by comprehensive revision and need 'shoring up' before they can be utilised well to support new behaviours.

8. Guilt, in Kellyan terminology, describes an awareness that a person is behaving out of their usual role. It is of course strongly bound up with the above points and probably explains the reluctance of people who stutter to maintain techniques of fluency, which are so easy to attain. Countless people who stutter complain they do not feel normal or natural, sound odd and would, quite honestly, prefer to stutter. Donning fluency implies putting on an act and the person has little or no system with which to construe the event. It is an intriguing paradox that the person who stutters feels guilty when she does so because she is acting out of the role she has for herself when not speaking and also feels guilty when she is fluent. This does not feel normal either and reactions are hard to predict.

9. Possibly the single most important and treacherous phenomenon common to the majority of people who stutter both mildly and severely is that of avoidance. This is the act of postponement, the changing of one sound for another or one word for another, choosing not to enter a situation or choosing not to be something on account of stuttering. Sheehan (1970) described five different levels of avoidance including sound, word, situation, relationship and even self. Avoidance has been described by people who stutter as their only 'technique' for not stuttering, the reason given being related to a feeling of panic, a strong desire neither to have the feelings that accompany stuttering nor to be seen stuttering. They feel out of control and they feel as if their listener is reacting negatively. They also say, however, that the act of avoidance itself leaves an extremely negative feeling of failure and a sense of frustration. The problem and all that goes with it has not changed for the better. It has simply been concealed.

The reasons behind avoidance may be many and varied. It may be considered, for example, to be an act of Kellyan hostility. It has already been stated that the person who stutters understands their world best through the elaborated construct system of stuttering. Whilst this may indeed be a 'poor implement' it is the most elaborate and consistent they have and the need to have predictions validated is powerful. It may be necessary to 'extort validational evidence of a type which supports predictions'. The states of anxiety and threat aroused by unpredictability probably contribute greatly to the need to withdraw from a situation. At first, this act of withdrawal from, for example, a word or a situation, produces relief in that the need for prediction about the speech act is eliminated but, if reality is never tested, soon the individual starts to wonder what would have happened and to resent the loss of control. Guilt, anxiety and threat once again set in, reinforced as the person feels frustrated by the lack of choice about what to say and when. This is only made worse when stuttering re-emerges following avoidance tactics. Once again predictions are unstable in that now avoidance may or may not precede stuttering. It may be true to say that the construct 'stuttering' is consistently invalidated as a tool for effective communication overall, as described by Kelly when discussing the notion of 'disorder', but it may be the only available tool for predicting how the experiment of a communicative interchange will go. Avoidance is certainly not a better alternative and simply fuels the 'pump of fear' (Sheehan, 1970).

10. There may be issues about dependency reaching back to childhood indicating the operation of poorly elaborated pre-verbal constructs.

11. Employment and entertainment may have been selected with stuttering very much in mind, indicating the extent to which a person's world may be constricted.

Terms such as avoidance, expectancy, fear, shame, guilt, anxiety, embarrassment and frustration among others have been used by people who stutter to describe how they feel. Seen through the eyes of personal construct theory as some have been above, the problem is at once clearer and yet more complex. The therapist is aware that the predictive efficiency of the system does not allow optimum functioning but the dimensions along which changes could be made are many and varied. One thing does seem clear, however. Simple behavioural changes in the absence of reconstruction are inadvisable and will probably be resisted because the implications for change they will have for other parts of that person's system are too far reaching.

Views from Both Sides

The sociality corollary states that 'to the extent that one person construes the construction process of another, he or she may play a role in a social process involving the other person'. This act of attempting to view things from the other person's point of view is one which we are all conscious of doing sometimes well and sometimes badly. An examination of how the dysfluent speaker views the fluent speaker and vice versa underlines how far reaching poor execution of 'sociality' can be. If people who are uninformed about stuttering and who do not stutter themselves are asked about the phenomenon, it seems that they do have some constructs but that these tend to be constellatory or pre-emptive in nature; certainly unelaborated. They may focus on the words 'anxious', 'shy' or even 'brave' to describe someone who stutters but it can surprise the stuttering individual to find how anxious and threatened fluent speakers themselves are and how worried they are about how they are being perceived by the person who stutters. The adage 'You wouldn't worry about how much people thought about you if you knew how little they thought about you' may be uncomfortably true for both parties. The reason non-stutterers may avoid eye-contact first, laugh or respond 'wrongly' in some other way is usually because the event is lying outside the range of convenience of their construct system and they are anxious. Not only do they have a poorly elaborated system around the stuttering pole of 'fluency–stuttering' but this construct is unlikely to have discriminatory value at all for them. The person who stutters is again surprised to find that the phenomenon of stuttering has no place at all in the non-stutterer's construct system and is, in effect, uninteresting! The non-stutterer (unaware of his label at all) is also unable to predict the situation and must borrow constructs from other parts of experience to make sense of the event. Interaction, therefore, is often short and the communication is unrewarding, giving no support to the attempts nor validation to the experience for either party. It is probably not until both begin to construe the construction processes of the other that true communication will take place. Not only does this imply necessary dilation of constructs for the person who stutters but also education and a widening of perceptions for the general public. Research (Woods and Williams, 1976; Turnbaugh *et al.*, 1979; Silverman, 1982; Kalinowski and Watt, 1987) has shown that many different groups, even speech pathologists, have negative stereotypes of people who stutter and the media often portray the phenomenon through the medium of comedy rather than documentary, tragedy or as part of the normal cross-section of society, a goal sought by many other minority groups. The development of more propositional construing would be welcome indeed.

How people who stutter view non-stutterers is reflected in the whole chapter. If fluency is submerged and poorly elaborated and the whole construct system evolves tightly around stuttering, people who do not do it will be seen rather one-dimensionally. Fransella (1972) made the salutary observation that a client's reluctance to enter therapy was not surprising when you saw his construal of stutterers as good and fluent people as bad.

Personal Construct Therapy for People who Stutter

Just occasionally it becomes apparent that the application of personal construct theory to the actual treatment of stuttering has been misunderstood and needs clarification. By describing a client's therapy as 'doing PCT' – a common enough shorthand – the implication could be that it can stand by itself as a sort of curative technique. The way PCT is described in the literature does not usually focus on the stuttering behaviour *per se* but more on the effects of stuttering and change on the person as a whole. Not surprisingly, therefore, it can seem that the speech problem itself is being ignored in favour of discussion about feelings and attitudes. One of the main aims of this chapter is to elucidate (for therapists and clients) what a PCT approach to stuttering means. As stated before, it does not stand isolated as a form of therapy itself, but is a framework which subsumes other indicated procedures or techniques. In his article 'Behaviour is an experiment' (1970) Kelly presented this most powerfully. He stated that it can only be by doing something differently that we can ever start to change. However, it cannot simply be just the doing that creates the change. We have to be ready to accommodate those changes into our system and without this readiness no reconstruction will take place. The experience corollary and the notion of permeability explain this accommodation further and to exemplify it we only need ask one of the many people who stutter why they do not continue to use a speech technique such as prolonged speech which they learned to use very successfully during a week's intensive course at some time in the past. The answer may possibly be 'It sounded odd', or 'It didn't feel like me'. In other words, the change was seen purely as an act and no deeper reconstruction had taken place to provide a foundation for understanding how the whole person could accommodate the new behaviour and make psychological sense of it.

PCT is not something which is selected for use with some clients but not with others. If found to be useful by the therapist, it becomes the framework through which all clients may be viewed. This does not mean that each of these people need discuss the theory itself, spend a great deal of time probing into their feelings, nor complete a self-characterisation or grid. It may be best for the therapist to instruct a client only in the use of a speech technique such as prolonged speech because, at that point, this has been established as the best route towards change and reconstruction for this person. In the author's opinion, neither PCT nor behavioural techniques should be worked on in isolation. Without reconstruction, change will be short-lived and meaningless and without experimentation with behaviour change there will be nothing to reconstrue.

Fransella and Dalton (1990) say about personal construct counselling that it is 'the process of understanding the client's construing of the world as seen through the eyes of personal construct theory and thereby, being in a position to facilitate the client's reconstruing of life and experience'. The personal construct counsellor has important skills which include taking the 'as if' stance, subsuming, suspension, credulous listening, observation and creativity. These are achieved through the use of professional constructs described earlier. The speech and language therapist adds to this by making techniques of specific behaviour change known to enhance fluency available to the individual.

The Process of Therapy

This section will address the need to tailor therapy for the individual. The reason this may not always have happened in the past may be because the obvious similarities in stuttering behaviour have deceived us into believing that the people who stutter have identical problems. Whilst little variation in describable stuttering behaviour *per se* is actually possible physiologically, people tend to present with unique combinations of these behaviours and research by Beech and Fransella (1968) also shows us that people who stutter do not have similar personality traits. It seems that the underlying route each individual takes in becoming 'someone who stutters' is invariably confusingly different and the content of their construct systems is not alike. Because the routes taken in the development of stuttering and the nature of each person's stuttering are so different surely it must be inappropriate to treat people who stutter with similar therapies? Therapy which looks at an individual's system of construing, identifies the degree and direction of behavioural change, locates impedance to change and which is able to encourage reconstruing is usually more successful than treatment of the symptom alone. Not only does it select really meaningful and well-timed movements but also encourages the development of the therapeutic alliance between therapist and client as a true partnership. This type of approach to therapy is not unique and may be found in the work of Watzlawick *et al.* in 1974 (described in more detail in Hayhow's chapter within this volume) who explain the way second-order change (therapist and client reframe the problem) is more effective than first-order change which concentrates on the symptoms of the problem.

At the risk of being dogmatic a flow chart of therapy for the adult who stutters is proposed, as shown in Figure 7.1.

In many ways such a flow chart is most unsatisfactory because it leaves so much unsaid and fails even to raise a number of issues. In other ways it is valuable because it underlines the fact that decisions about the best form of therapy draw on numerous, complex factors and needs to accommodate the changing levels within each area and, consequently, the changing person as a whole. If, however, the client can share the burden of decision making and understand the variables involved to a relevant degree it is felt that they will understand the aims of therapy better and obtain greater benefit from the process.

The initial meeting with each person who stutters only serves to underline the point that stuttering is a very heterogeneous disorder and that all clients are very different. The personal philosophy behind PCT is immediately useful in that it prevents the therapist from becoming judgemental and stereotyping. In the author's experience, it is very rare to find any two people responding in a similar fashion to their difficulties and, without the security of observing this through a framework, it would have been difficult to take on board. It may be that the inability to carry out technique-based programmes with people who stutter successfully without tailoring them personally for each client may be at the root of much therapist anxiety about treating stuttering.

The bones of the theory as described previously are utilised by the therapist in making a transitive diagnosis with the client. Assessment of stuttering traditionally consists of speech profile information and attitude questionnaires, thus supplying both overt and covert stuttering information. In order to ensure that these tools are doing more than observing the extent to which the current client fits in with the therapist's stereotype of stuttering, it is vital to find out other important information which might influence change. Knowledge about the client's content and structure of construing is gained from a number of different methods including structured interview, laddering, pyramiding and self-characterisation, all described in detail in the texts suggested previously. A number of grid methods are currently available including the repertory grid, the implications grid and the dependency grid. Whilst the use

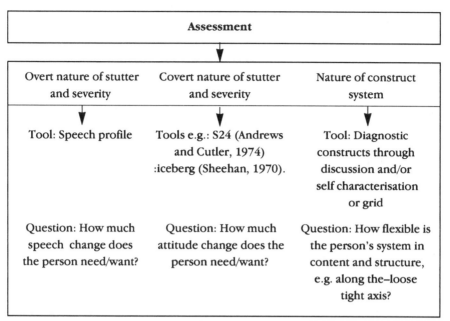

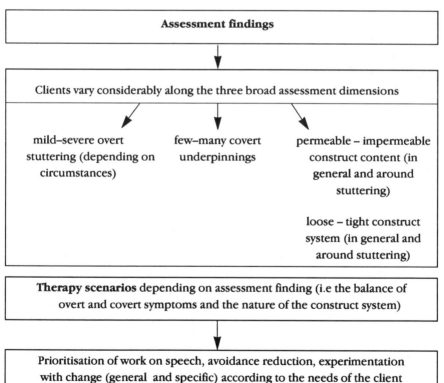

Figure 7.1 Flow chart of therapy for the adult stutterer

of these is not obligatory, it can be extremely useful with many clients in allowing the therapist to subsume the client's system quickly and in focusing on work to be done.

Kelly's first principle of assessment – 'ask the client what the problem is, he may just tell you' – has immediate appeal, and is possibly best applied through his tool of the 'self-characterisation'. Even here, variation between clients is remarkable, supporting the notion that often the time spent doing an 'assessment' is as important as the result or even more so. For example, one client spent approximately six sessions using her self-characterisation as a basis for weekly discussion as she was surprised and concerned with the content of a large number of constructs. Another found that the experience of writing it was a more holistic experience and his interest lay in viewing the structure of his system. This 'assessment method', therefore, led the way for therapy in that one therapeutic process initially involved examination of content, and the other of structure. This is not to say that this was the only form of therapy indicated but it was initially meaningful for the client and provided a non-threatening and satisfying area in which to experiment.

Assessment is seen as an ongoing experiment which upholds the PCT philosophy of 'person-as-scientist'. Clients contribute greatly to their own assessment and where he or she construes stuttering symptomatically and has a relatively tight system around frequency and duration of blocks it may be important in the first instance to assess this and use symptom-based therapy. This does not mean to say that no attempt should be made to dilate their view in order to introduce the other positive aspects of communication. Symptom-based assessment and therapy is rooted firmly in the philosophy of PCT where it provides a basis for reconstruction.

Therapy is, therefore, a continuation of the transitive diagnosis and is seen as a reframing of the problem following careful examination of the individual, planning for future experiments and reconstruction. Any form can be used which is appropriate for the stuttering client and may be attitude- or symptom-based or some of each. What is important is that it should be seen as experimenting with change and viewed as the opportunity to reconstrue. It will probably involve most or all the dimensions of transition and, if there is experimentation with fluency, this will need to be sensitively done for it to be incorporated eventually into the person's construct system. Unless change takes place and is accepted on more than the 'fluent–stuttering' axis, the person who stutters will remain in the age-old dilemma of slot rattling because the new system is insufficiently elaborated, cannot generalise and just plain does not fit! Some clients have in fact left therapy having found that they were unhappy with any form of change and that, at least for the present, the old construct system was one they wished to continue to use. Rather surprisingly for the inexperienced author at that time, this outcome was a positive one for one client who, having investigated alternatives, found them not to be constructive and went off happy! It may be, however, that the very occurrence of his open, 'aggressive', investigation would, in the future, initiate changes which he would be able to incorporate slowly and carefully.

The value of using professional constructs was highlighted recently when a client began to resist doing any work at home in preparation for her sessions and she and the therapist were both aware of the need to look for a more fundamental and important reason than laziness! The process of change was examined from the point when the client had started personal construct therapy for her stutter a year previously with another therapist, had been enlightened and pleased with new insights, and had incorporated some changes, definitely loosening a tight system. The therapist then left, the client had respite from contact but six months later got in touch with the author. She wanted to continue with personal construct therapy and showed great enthusiasm for change and the acceptance of herself as someone who stuttered. From aspects of the self-characterisation, the fact that the client was experimenting with a drama class and that she was actively seeking alternatives, the process of loosening was continued even to the extent of examining 'blocking' behaviour through visual imagery as if it were a dream sequence. For some time the client was fascinated and her insights were having a beneficial effect on her life, allowing her to view friends less narrowly and reduce anxiety. Then, within the space of a few weeks, anxiety increased and 'homework', which involved exercises in alternative reconstruing and loosening, was resisted.

At the time of first entering therapy the client was leading a predictable life; continuing with her PhD and not involved in an emotional relationship. During the latter stages of therapy the PhD was coming to a close and she was faced with a novel experience – not having her academic career carved out for her. She had also begun a serious emotional attachment. It was obvious, therefore, that not only was her lifestyle beginning to be unpredictable but that her new looser style of construing events was not yet strong enough to support so much change all at once. It was decided that therapy should focus on 'tighter' elements, especially the here and now, and initially a repertory grid was set up. This tightening phase of the creativity cycle was supportive and changes were maintained. It is possible that the alternative may have been a swift 'slot rattle' back to old systems. During the discussions, however, an interesting and profound implicative dilemma was discovered using Tschudi's (1977) ABC model. The client stated that her real fear was to be 'out of control' whilst being 'in control' was preferred. When asked about the advantages of ' being out of control' these were described as 'taking active responsibilities for your actions' and 'approaching life positively' – something the client had set up as an aim!.

Conversely, the disadvantage of being 'in control' was 'passive acceptance of what happens'. Once insight was gained here and the threat of
change was addressed more fully, the client's constructs became more
permeable and she could look at the dilemma with some interest and
begin to reconstrue, initially through the devising of different verbal
labels. Hayhow and Levy (1989) describe how therapy tries to 'help a
client evolve a construct system through which they can move towards
their objectives' where optimal functioning is the goal. Professional
constructs support both the client's and the therapist's insight into this
process.

Change

Therapy for people who stutter is most particularly about the possibilities there may be for change. However, no change is simple, and the
person involved must constantly balance the degree of aggression
(active elaboration of one's perceptual field) they can afford against the
degree of anxiety and threat aroused by any proposed elaboration.
Change involves complex patterns of decision making and, sometimes,
facing up to unexpected consequences. Buscaglia (1982) suggested that
there are three requirements for change:

(a) the individual should be dissatisfied with him- or herself;
(b) there should be a conscious decision to change; and
(c) there must be a conscious dedication to the process of growth and
    change.

The first two are expressed relatively easily but the third is often
extremely difficult to achieve. Maybe this 'conscious dedication' is only
possible if the alteration of a speech pattern is made part of the person
as a whole instead of something used when apparently needed (imply-
ing that stuttering has still not been fully accepted). There is a level of
commitment to change, either behavioural or attitudinal, which has a
'wholehearted' feel about it. The content of a person's constructs and
his or her system has somehow balanced the part stuttering has to play
so that it has become something that they do rather than something that
they are. Such comprehensive change involving core constructs obviously will not have been quick or easy. Neither will it imply the same
result for each person. Some individuals achieve a high degree of fluency
using a technique, others modify their stuttering to an easier form and
still more remain with a residual stutter.

'Using' PCT might be seen as 'not so much a therapy, more a way of
life' to borrow part of one of Fransella's memorable statements from
1970. For therapists, assistance is given in, first, moving through very
muddy waters and, second, in recognising their own anxiety as a very
natural phenomenon. Because of its reflexivity the theory helps the ther-

apist to understand the process and provides a construct system of its own for clarifying difficult issues. Whilst change must take place for the client, the therapist is also undergoing revisions of constructs, and by preventing or resisting this a sterile environment is likely to develop. Fransella notes that change is possible only when we have some understanding of where we are going, which is why the transitive diagnosis is imperative.

The principle of constructive alternativism allows the client and the therapist the possibility of exploring numerous changes. As part of the credulous approach the therapist must not only be aware that such changes have serious implications for many parts of the client's system, but also that they vary along several rather obvious but sometimes obscured dimensions. Some of these include:

- Time: some changes need longer than others. The client's time scale is often different from the therapist's.
- Quality: changes which seem great to the client may not seem so to the therapist, or to the people near to the person who stutters.
- Quantity: people have differing needs in the numbers of changes they can accommodate at any one time.
- Saliency: the importance of the change needs to be seen from the viewpoint of the client and this can be missed by the therapist.
- Contingency changes: some changes cannot take place until others have already been addressed. For example, a client may have an extremely tight, pre-emptive construct system where most of his predictions relate strongly to his constructs about stuttering. Further discussion reveals that he finds the prospect of 'being wrong' threatening and anxiety producing. It is clear that unless this second factor is reconstrued more usefully the client will get nowhere with the first.
- Changes as consequences: the awareness that other changes will naturally follow the first.

Why no Change?

Resistance to change is described vividly by Fransella (1972) through the choice corollary. The person chooses to remain 'a stutterer' because it is from this view that he has the greatest extension and elaboration of his system. He understands himself better and feels he can predict in spite of these predictions, in one sense, being constantly invalidated. Where fluency is attempted or constructs are overhauled, it may be that the implicative dilemmas are too great to allow change at what may be a subordinate level or that the loosening of a person's system which may be necessary to accommodate fluency into it may generate a wholesale loosening which is actually dangerous for the client.

Aggressive change on the positive poles, before they are fully elaborated, leads to impulsivity followed by hostility. Sometimes the client is so enthusiastic about new-found fluency he does not give himself time to elaborate the underpinning constructs.

Even clients, however, who appear to have responded to new insights with admirable experimentation and skill and who have committed themselves wholeheartedly to speech modification are left with residual stuttering behaviour. It seems rare to find someone who considers themselves an 'ex-stutterer' and it may be that a constitutional component of stuttering is involved.

It is unusual for there to have been no change at all in a client and, in order to be lasting, time should be given for comprehensive alterations to be absorbed into the system as a whole. In other words, the idea of 'why no change?' may be misplaced. Fluency, to whatever degree, must be allowed to feel comfortable and familiar. Sometimes changes on too many fronts are contra-indicated or resisted by the client and need not be seen as failure by the client or the therapist.

Evaluation of Therapy

Evaluation of therapy remains a difficult issue in that if a simple quantitative measure is not used to begin with then we cannot reassess using it either. Also, if therapy does not prescribe 100% fluency as the intended outcome, quantitative measures are less useful. Within the framework of PCT, the therapist utilises diagnostic or professional constructs to gain a picture and periodically reviews the areas covered with the client. Systems do not accommodate change or fluency in a convenient 'growth-curve' fashion and it is usual for people who stutter to fluctuate in their stuttering frequency as well as their mood and attitude at different times. Whether it is possible to assess whether therapy was responsible for significant change is always hard and especially so when change is sought on such a wide variety of levels. If, however, the dimensions of, for example, 'tight–loose construing' or 'pre-emptive–propositional construing' are being used, then descriptive objectivity is possible. Another estimation of the effectiveness of therapy must also be the degree of client satisfaction, again difficult to quantify but certainly possible to estimate. One study using measurement of fluency was by Evesham and Fransella (1985) who found that relapse was reduced in clients who were encouraged to elaborate the meaningfulness of fluency at the same time as using a speech technique.

Reconstruction is probably impossible piecemeal, and is obviously very difficult to measure. Although the ultimate aim of stuttering therapy must be to reduce the disfluency, this is only valid if it makes the person feel better. If it does not, as in the case of unaccommodated behavioural change, the fact that the frequency of stuttering moments is reduced is rendered meaningless. The act itself is a symptom which Kelly described as 'simply the meaning a person has given to otherwise chaotic experiences'. If therapy involves the development of meaning and the restructuring of these 'chaotic experiences', then change must be measured within the construct system, not just through the outward expression. What people say about their stuttering, either through grids, self-characterisations or in conversation, as well as the evidence of reduced avoidance and acknowledgement of stuttering, must indicate if a system is, for example, less tightly structured round a symptom or is more permeable.

Current research by Enderby (in process) utilises the World Health Organisation's labels of 'impairment', 'disability' and 'handicap' and adds 'distress/well-being' to describe the effect of therapeutic intervention on client groups (including people who stutter) where change is so difficult to measure. Early figures already show that whilst percentage change is not clear in the impairment (the neuropsychological and neurophysiological events which accompany the audible and visible manifestations of stuttering behaviour), there are some changes in the disability (the audible and visible manifestations of stuttering) and there is often a powerful effect of therapy on the parameters of handicap and, especially, distress/well-being. In other words, in spite of residual stuttering, the person has changed with respect to socialisation, their job prospects and their sense of self-worth. Curlee (1993) stresses the usefulness of this model in framing the problem but adds how difficult it is to measure the handicap.

Conclusion

PCT is a theory of personality and as such provides a structure for understanding people and occasionally their problems. The theory can be shared with clients and applies equally usefully to the therapist and the process of therapy. This means that traditional methods that speech and language therapists employ to facilitate fluency in their clients may be highly relevant but need careful selection in order to make them useful for the individual. Finally, PCT is not something the person who stutters is given or undergoes!. What they do is experiment with symptom and/or attitude change and then reconstrue.

References

Andrews, G. and Cutler, J. (1974). The relationship between changes in symptom level and attitude. *Journal of Speech and Hearing Disorders* 39, 312–319.

Beech, H.R. and Fransella, F. (1968). *Research and Experiment in Stuttering*. New York: Pergamon.

Bloodstein, O. (1975). 'Stuttering as tension and fragmentation'. In: Eisenson, J. (Ed.), *Stuttering: a Second Symposium*. New York: Harper & Row.

Buscaglia, L. (1982). *Love*. New York: Fawcett Crest.

Curlee, R. and Perkins, W. (1985). *The Nature and Treatment of Stuttering*. London: Taylor & Francis.

Curlee, R.F. (1993). Evaluating treatment efficacy for adults: assessment of stuttering disability. *Journal of Fluency Disorders* **18**, 319–331.

Dalton, P. (1983). Psychological approaches to the treatment of stuttering. In: Dalton, P. (Ed.), *Approaches to the Treatment of Stuttering*. Beckenham: Croom Helm.

Dalton, P. (1994). *Counselling People with Communication Problems*. London: Sage.

Dalton, P. and Dunnett, G. (1992). *A Psychology for Living: Personal Construct Theory for Professionals and Clients*. Chichester: Wiley.

Enderby, P. (1992). Outcome measures in speech therapy: Impairment, disability, handicap and distress. *Health Trends* **24**(2).

Evesham, M. and Fransella, F. (1985). Stuttering relapse: the effect of a combined speech psychological reconstruction programme. *British Journal of Disorders of Communication* **20**, 237–248.

Fransella, F. (1970). Stuttering: not a symptom but a way of life. *British Journal of Disorders of Communication* **5**, 20–29.

Fransella, F. (1972). *Personal Change and Reconstruction*. London: Academic Press.

Fransella, F. and Dalton, P. (1990). *Personal Construct Counselling in Action* London: Sage.

Hayhow, R. and Levy, C. (1989). *Working with Stuttering: A Personal Construct Therapy Approach*. Oxford: Winslow Press.

Kalinowski, J.S. and Watt, J. (1987). A preliminary examination of the perceptions of self and others in stutterers and non-stutterers. *Journal of Fluency Disorders* **12**, 317–331.

Kelly, G.A. (1955). *The Psychology of Personal Constructs*, Vols 1 and 2. New York: Norton.

Kelly, G.A. (1970). Behaviour is an experiment. In: D. Bannister (Ed.), *Perspectives in Personal Construct Theory*. London and New York: Academic Press.

Leitner, L.M. (1981). Psychopathology and the differentiation of values, emotions and behaviours: a repertory grid study. *British Journal of Psychiatry* **138**, 147–153.

Prins, D. (1993) Models for treatment efficacy: studies of adult stutterers. *Journal of Fluency Disorders* **18**, 339–349.

Sheehan, J. (1970). *Stuttering: Research and Therapy*. New York: Harper & Row.

Silverman, E.M. (1982). Speech-language clinicians' and university students' impressions of women and girls who stutter. *Journal of Fluency Disorders* **7**, 469–478.

Starkweather, W. (1987). *Fluency and Stuttering*. Englewood Cliffs, NJ: Prentice-Hall.

Tschudi, F. (1977). Loaded and honest questions: a construct theory view of symptoms and therapy. In: D. Bannister (Ed.), *New perspectives in Personal Construct Theory*. London: Academic Press.

Turnbaugh, K.R., Guitar, B.E. and Hoffman, P.R. (1979). Speech Clinicians' attribution of personality traits as a function of stuttering severity. *Journal of Speech and Hearing Research*, **22**, 37–45.

Van Riper, C. (1982). *The Nature of Stuttering*. Englewood Cliffs, NJ: Prentice-Hall.

Watzlawick, P., Weakland, J. and Fisch, R. (1974). *Change: Principles of Problem Formation and Problem Resolution*. New York: Norton.

Winter, D.A .(1992). *Personal Construct Psychology in Clinical Practice: Theory, Research and Application*. London: Routledge.

Woods, C.L. and Williams, D.E. (1976). Traits attributed to stuttering and normally fluent males. *Journal of Speech and Hearing Research* **19**, 267–279.

Chapter 8
Qualities of the Therapist: Implications for Student Training

RENEE BYRNE

> We can become all the clinician we can become as long as we realize that we are the ones who have to do the becoming.
>
> (Conture, 1990)

This statement may contain one of the most important functions of training: that students understand educators can teach, help, advise and cajole, but it is the student who must do the 'becoming'.

In this chapter emphasis will be placed on undergraduate training because it is at this stage that important, long-term concepts are formed; 'attitudes that are strongly held are more likely than not to be retained throughout a lifetime' (Leahy, 1994). The student is influenced in the acquisition of basic beliefs, learns to evaluate issues, goes through a process of growth and self-awareness, begins to see him- or herself as a certain kind of clinician, wants to work with some disorders and not with others. Various issues will be raised which may continue to generate interest amongst educators, clinicians and students.

Does the Stutterers' Therapist require Special Skills?

In a Utopian world, clinicians would have every attribute required for treating all conditions. Since we do not live in Utopia, it would seem that the stutterers' therapist does require certain specific skills.

Stuttering presents the student with many controversies, copious literature, contradictory research data, and some conflicting theories. 'Stuttering remains an enigma in spite of the fact that it has been studied, at some level, for centuries. More has been written about stuttering than about any other disorders of speech, yet it is still less well understood than the others. In no small measure the reason stuttering is so poorly understood is because so much has been written about it; the intrinsic mystery of the disorder has been embellished by the many efforts to explain it' (Wingate, 1988).

Students and therapists frequently complain that they are confused by the presentation of differing aetiologies, theories and therapeutic approaches related to stuttering. This confusion can lead to clinicians feeling inadequate when dealing with children and adults who stutter. Training at undergraduate level must aim to keep the subject clear and unthreatening so that students are eager to work with stutterers and feel competent and confident to do so.

Gregory (1978) defined two major categories in therapy, the 'speak-more-fluently' and the 'stutter-more-fluently' approaches. Using this categorisation, it is possible to allay students' anxieties about the vast number of techniques available for treating stutterers because most procedures can be classified under one or other of these two major headings. It is important for students to understand the pros and cons of approaches, and to understand that techniques are not mutually exclusive, but can be combined. Students can become anxious about whether a 'speak-more-fluently' or a stutter-more-fluently' approach should be used when treating specific clients, but this is putting the cart before the horse. If a child or adult is referred as being 'a stutterer' this is not sufficiently descriptive, and careful assessment procedures should be utilised to acquire sufficient information in order to answer the question, 'How can this client be helped?'. Confusion, relating to choice of approaches, can be minimised for students if they begin to realise that it is only after that question is answered that a decision can be made as to which initial therapeutic approach is most suitable.

Therapists and students seek to feel secure in the knowledge that they are using the 'right' approach. Too frequently, students believe that they must know the exact procedure to follow as soon as the child or adult enters the clinic room. Stuttering is a complex, multifaceted problem and there is no single, simplistic cure; also, stuttering is not a homogeneous disorder, nor is it solely a speech problem because psycho-social, neuro-physiological and personality features must be considered. Therefore, students need to understand that careful assessment and the formation of a trusting relationship with the client and/or parent is part of treatment and not an aspect that should be quickly completed before 'proper' therapy can be instituted. Training must stress this aspect so that the student does not feel pressurised to implement one or other therapeutic technique before the stutterer and his/her problem is adequately understood. The student should feel comfortable taking a case history, considering ongoing assessment, and allowing time for discussion of the issues involved in therapy.

A second point for consideration is that stutterers are not 'ill' and cannot be viewed as 'patients' so that their relationship with the clinician differs from that which can be formed with many other client groups. The majority of a clinician's workload involves a patient–therapist relationship which must exist primarily on an instructional basis because the patient is a child, who requires 'teaching', or an adult who is incapacitated in one way or another. In the case of an adult stutterer, or the parent of a child who stutters, the clinician is dealing with a healthy human being who happens to have a speech problem, or with the parent of a child who has a speech problem.

Frequently, the client is of a similar age to the therapist, and the relationship the therapist may need to form will be of a non-instructional, inter-personal partnership. In training, tutors will be sensitive to the fact that students can feel deeply threatened because they are required to form a more exposing relationship than may occur with an 'ill' patient. Adult stutterers and the parents of stutterers can, and do, answer back, express emotions, criticise the student and refute suggestions offered. In order to train the effective stutterers' therapist, it is advisable to consider including in the syllabus a significant section devoted to training student self-awareness and self-development rather than viewing this aspect as peripheral to academic factors in the degree course.

During the past couple of decades there has been a considerable shift of emphasis in many disciplines, and certainly in the field of stuttering therapy. Kanfer (1980) terms this a shift from an administrative to a participant model of treatment. Therapists no longer see their role as advising or instructing the client what to do whilst the client plays a somewhat passive role; rather, in the participant model, great stress is laid on the client taking equal responsibility with the therapist for the course of treatment and for the maintenance of improvement. This change in emphasis has necessitated a parallel change in the training of therapists. Attention has become focused on the learning of self-management and problem-solving approaches in order that clients can be helped to implement such approaches – regardless of the therapeutic technique offered.

What Knowledge is Needed by the Therapist Working with People Who Stutter?

In order to discuss training, criteria are required as to the aims of such training: what is the student to become or acquire? Hopefully, the issues and topics discussed in this chapter will help towards answering the question.

An adequate theoretical and academic framework is necessary because, without this, clinical intervention would have no concrete foundation. Arguably, of equal significance is the acquisition of intra- and inter-personal skills because, without these, the essential client–therapist relationship can break down; also, some understanding of the psychological processes that may help to maintain stuttering in certain clients is thought by many to be essential. In an age of scarce resources, treatment evaluation and the collection of outcome data must be an important part of training.

Conflicts arise as to whether students should be taught to be eclectic in approach or more specific. Hayhow and Levy (1989) state that 'it is important for therapists to have a clear theoretical framework upon which to base their work....so that we are not forced into a position of eclectics...'. Whereas Conture (1990) says, 'The idea that stuttering should be treated either this way or that way is very much related, we think, to our "t'is-t'aint" views of what causes stuttering....Typically, the battle lines have been drawn between psyche (essentially a nurture idea) and the soma (essentially a nature idea). Both approaches have some validity, but neither, by itself, appears sufficient'. In training, clarity is required on this and other conflicting issues before a sensible programme can be devised.

Stuttering is often seen by therapists and students as something 'different', and educators can help their students to learn that skills in one area of speech pathology can, and should, be transferred to other areas. A student who, on meeting a six-year-old stutterer, tells the tutor that she cannot deal with this child because she has never seen a six-year-old stutterer before, has not learnt that a six-year-old child, although possessing unique qualities, will still be a six-year-old child whether the child has a stutter, language delay or a phonological disorder. The student should be helped to see the child first and the speech problem second rather than vice versa. It is known that a significant number of children who show signs of disfluencies have articulatory and/or language problems (Dalton and Hardcastle, 1990; Conture, 1990). Stuttering can be an emotive topic for parents, teachers and clinicians so that this condition can mask other difficulties such as hearing loss, emotional problems, dyslexia and so forth. Therefore, although issues specific to stuttering are important in training, it is also essential for students to understand that stuttering requires the same careful, global assessment and diagnosis as other speech disorders.

Many children, adolescents and adults are seen in groups either intensively or on a weekly basis and, therefore, theoretical and experiential work in this area is valuable.

Parents are now considered an integral part of most speech and language therapy with children but, in the treatment and management of disfluent children, parents are often asked to implement management programmes, and the child may well not be seen in the clinic after the initial interview. This requires a trusting relationship with the parents, counselling skills, and an ability to offer advice and give information. Although some of this work will be done when learning about other child client groups, it is frequently necessary to help students gain confidence when working solely through parents.

How Important is the Therapist's Role in the Treatment of Stutterers?

In 1975 Van Riper wrote, 'Millions of words have been written about stutterers, but only a few about the clinicians who treat them. Surely it is time to examine stuttering therapy from this other perspective. No matter what kind of treatment is used and no matter what its rationale may be the clinician is always a significant part of the therapeutic triad.' Murphy and Fitzsimmons (1960) put the situation more succinctly with, 'the most important single variable in success in the treatment of stutterers is – the clinician'. Most would agree with Van Riper that the 'clinician is always a significant part of the therapeutic triad', but the situation becomes more controversial when it is claimed that the clinician is the single most important variable in successful outcome. Further research is needed to establish the importance of the client–clinician relationship in the successful outcome of stuttering therapy, and to assess clinicians' attitudes, characteristics and personalities which may be of significance.

There is countless anecdotal evidence to the effect that a certain technique proved efficacious for a client when administered by therapist B, but was of little value when administered by therapist A. However, the equation in stuttering is not so simple. Questions need to be asked such as: When did therapist A offer this technique? Was the client more mature, more receptive when therapist B came on the scene? What was going on in the rest of the client's life when therapy was administered by A and B? Did the client have more realistic expectations of therapy when encountering therapist B? It is extremely difficult to separate the qualities of the therapist from the type of therapy offered and the receptiveness of the client. However, few would argue that the clinician is of considerable import in the successful management of a client.

Many authorities have tried to define the personal attributes required by the therapist, and certain qualities have been identified. Cooper (1966) and Cooper *et al.* (1971) used various personality scales to rate clinicians on two parameters: a student–teacher instructional basis and a clinician–client non-instructional parameter. The studies showed that the effective clinician tended to express control over others, wanted to be included in activities by others, and needed to express and receive affection. Schriberg *et al.* (1977) summarised their findings by stating that the better clinicians tend to have an internal locus of control and, perhaps, a higher fear of disapproval, whilst the poorer clinicians tend to have a higher need to appear good and have more emotional instability. Haynes and Oratio (1978) noted, 'Our data indicate that from the adult client's perspective, the establishment of an empathetic, genuine interpersonal relationship appears to be a good therapeutic investment. Speech-language pathologists should develop skills specific to the interpersonal dimensions and not be reticent about exhibiting their own personalities as opposed to 'playing the role' of a clinician. This seems to be an important factor, and of particular relevance in the training of clinicians.

The question of 'role-playing' or, conversely, the honesty of the clinician is frequently mentioned in the relevant literature. I learnt my lesson many years ago at a time when clinicians still wore white coats and tended to think that there was a particular, stereotypical therapist's role that had to be achieved. This role included being calm, cool and collected at all times, showing little or no emotion and never being confrontational. When I first qualified, I tried very hard to play this role, until one day a young woman with a stutter said, 'I can't work with you because you're not for real'. This was an entirely true statement but, in view of my 'role', it was difficult to decide how to respond: stay calm, cool and so forth, or be myself. I decided on the latter course since this young woman had obviously blown my cover. I explained quite honestly that, if I stopped being a 'perfect therapist', I might get bossy or challenging or critical or any of the things that she would not like and that I had been taught were professionally unacceptable. The young woman said, 'Please be yourself – at least it would be honest'. It is my belief that adults and children need honesty because it shows respect for them and is the only possible basis of a real therapeutic relationship.

Of course, there are other interpersonal skills that are generally found to be of importance and these might include an ability to:

- listen attentively;
- adapt treatment to the needs of the client on an ongoing basis;
- give information clearly and succinctly and make sure it is understood;
- convey optimism in the treatment offered and the ability of the client to implement the treatment;
- plan clear short- and long-term aims with space to deviate when necessary;
- refrain from interpretations and explanations which cause client confusion and increase complexity of the stuttering problem.

Counselling and Psychotherapy

'Since therapy with stuttering necessarily involves psychotherapy to some degree, it is not too much to ask of the clinician who would work with stutterers that he become reasonably knowledgeable on both subjects. A therapist with such twin knowledge is the best hope of the stutterer' (Sheehan, 1979). Specialist stuttering therapists frequently take a postgraduate training in counselling and, in the UK, Personal Construct Psychology has become closely linked with stuttering therapy

(Fransella, 1972; Hayhow and Levy, 1989; Dalton and Dunnett, 1990). Some degree of counselling training is included in most undergraduate speech and language courses but many would argue that there should be additional counselling training geared specifically to the problem of stuttering.

In this context, it is important to distinguish between a speech and language therapist using counselling skills as opposed to those working as counsellors. Students can learn counselling skills, and these will be useful in dealing with most client groups – skills such as selective listening, reflecting, facilitating and structuring can be acquired and practised during training.

Apart from these specific skills, the student needs to understand his/her own strengths and weaknesses, biases and prejudices. Without this knowledge, students can become qualified therapists and still feel threatened when clients become angry, aggressive, defensive, rejecting, accusatory and so forth. If the therapist believes that all these emotions are directed at him or her, then a defensive reaction can be displayed, and the overall aims of therapy will become obscured. Increasingly, it is becoming recognised that undergraduate programmes need to encompass some form of self-awareness training for students so that they are able to communicate with, and help, various client groups without finding that their own problems and prejudices come between them and the client. This type of training is useful when dealing with parents, other professionals, and most client groups. However, it may be important to take that training a little further when working with stuttering clients or their parents.

Clinicians' and Students' Prejudices

There is a body of research in this area, and it has been found that a significant percentage of students come to college with certain prejudices about stuttering and stutterers (St Louis and Lass,1981), and that training can sometimes strengthen rather than weaken these prejudices (Leahy, 1994). Clinicians' attitudes towards stuttering show that this is so (Woods and Williams, 1976), although it would seem that clinicians' attitudes are shifting (Cooper and Cooper, 1985). It has been noted that a similarity in attitudes was found between clinicians in the UK and those in the USA (Cooper and Rustin, 1985). Thus, research shows definite clinician bias and a far too frequent attitude of, 'Oh, I can't treat stutterers'! This attitude is then passed on to students during their clinical experience and again perpetuated by these students when qualified. It is something that can be borne in mind by educators when training the stutterers' therapist. On questioning clinicians and students it would seem that their anxieties fall into these main categories:

'I don't see many stutterers and so do not feel experienced' (usually quite true, but what about transferrable skills?).

'I hardly had any training at college regarding stuttering and stutterers' (can be true, but there are short postgraduate courses).

'The theory and practice of treating stutterers is so diffuse and complicated, I have no idea where to start' (partly true, but there are published programmes and books which are extremely helpful).

'Stutterers don't get better and can get worse during treatment' (not based on fact; many children are cured and adults can improve greatly).

If the above remarks are considered during training then many of these anxieties could be dispelled.

Some Ideas on Implementation

The majority of this chapter has been devoted to discussing various issues in training because it may be that, once the issues are identified, answers about implementation will follow. There are relatively few articles relating to the 'how's' of training students to work with people who stutter, and so a few ideas for discussion are offered. As has been mentioned, it is important that students gain an essential theoretical basis, and it is assumed that this is available to whatever extent is required by specific universities. However, it would seem equally important that students gain confidence in their own abilities, understand that skills learnt in one area can be transferred to another, and that stutterers are human beings. The student who leaves college with this type of awareness will be able to use his or her personal qualities and skills to implement theoretical knowledge in working with stuttering clients. It could be thought to be the job of educators to increase motivation and interest whilst decreasing prejudice and bias.

Data collected from the reports of both graduate and postgraduate students suggest that contact with people who stutter is an essential aspect of training, as this contact can serve 'to highlight both the effects upon a person's life and the different levels of stuttering that exist; also, this makes subsequent lectures more relevant' (taken from a student's report, 1994).

It is helpful to organise a number of tutorial sessions based on the work of Lay (1982) where students are encouraged to experiment with behavioural change, and begin to discover what this involves, as well as experiencing how groups function.

A certain amount of self-awareness can also be learnt in such tutorials. Experiential work of any kind seems invaluable in training and, although lectures and seminars are of importance, experiential work is effective in making such lectures relevant and in internalising issues for the students.

Students can be encouraged to try pseudo-stuttering and avoidance behaviours; work in this area will make them aware of some of the feelings experienced by stutterers. Slowed speech or slow-prolonged speech when practised on a hierarchical basis by students will do infinitely more to create awareness of difficulties in maintenance than will hours of lecturing.

There are major changes taking place both in the NHS and in the educational field, and there is no way of predicting the future clearly. At the time of writing, speech and language training is undertaken in universities and requires degree qualification. It could be that, in the future, candidates will take a first degree and speech and language therapy will be part of postgraduate training; or disorders of fluency may be removed from the general degree and form part of a postgraduate course. Increasingly, computer programmes will be utilised in training and clinical practice. Interactive programmes will be available to individual students in computer laboratories, or to tutorial groups with or without a tutor. For example, a split screen can show someone stuttering on one side whilst questions or comments are displayed on the other side of the screen. The trainee(s) can then interact with the computer at their own pace. Students will be trained in the use of voice-assisted systems so that they can help clients to employ these systems in the clinic. Such systems can be programmed for work on the more mechanical aspects of stuttering, such as breathing, rate control, tension and soft contacts.

Training cannot be viewed solely in terms of the initial qualification, but rather at various stages of the clinician's career there should be training appropriate to each stage. It is becoming increasingly important for clinicians to update and develop their skills throughout their career. Indeed, in order to maintain continuous registration with the College of Speech & Language Therapists, therapists pledge their commitment to further training.

Once the therapist has qualified, postgraduate, MSc and short courses, plus the possibility of an ACS (Advanced Clinical Studies Course), are all available training facilities.

A final comment: stuttering tends to be seen as the poor relation within the field of speech pathology. Lecturers, clinicians and students are urged to fight for an adequate share of time within the syllabus. Too often, academics and clinicians say, 'Oh well, it's just stuttering', but it is important for us all to remember that stuttering has been documented since the times of the early Greeks. It is probable that Moses stuttered, and Demosthenes certainly did. If it was a simple speech problem, a cure would have been found long ago. It is not a simple speech problem, but a complex, multifaceted disorder with mechanical speech, psychosocial, neuro-physiological, and psychological aspects. It is not a homogeneous disorder and as such we need more information about possible sub-groups or component factors. We now have finer assessment aids, scans, interactive computer analyses and so forth so that we are getting ever closer to understanding this complex problem, and the added knowledge should prove a challenge for interested parties to become involved through research, or clinically. There is a distinct possibility that, if stuttering were given more attention, it might reward those involved by yielding its secrets and thus bring us closer, not just to solving the riddle of stuttering but also to understanding far more about speech problems, and about the people who have speech problems. It is in training that it is possible to dispel negative attitudes about stuttering and stutterers and to motivate students, clinicians, academics and anyone who will listen to take an active interest in this fascinating subject.

References

Bloodstein, O. (1959). *Stuttering for Professional Workers*. Chicago: Easter Seal.
Brown, E. L.A. (1967). A university's approach to improving supervision. *Asha* 9, 476–479.
Byrne, R. (1991). *Let's Talk about Stammering*, 2nd edn. London: Association for Stammerers.
Byrne, R. and Jackson, M. (1984). Self-induced behavioural change: report on a student learning project. *Bulletin College of Speech Therapists* 391(November).
Conture, E.G. (1990). *Stuttering*, 2nd edn. New York: Prentice-Hall.
Cooper, E.B. (1966). Client–clinician relationship and concomitant factors in stuttering therapy. *Journal of Speech & Hearing Research* 9, 194–207.
Cooper, E.B. and Cooper, C. (1985). *Personalized Fluency Control Therapy*, revised edn. Hingham, MA: Teaching Resources.
Cooper, E.B. and Cooper, C.S. (1985). Clinician attitudes toward stuttering: a decade of change (1973–1983). *Journal of Fluency Disorders* 10, 19–33.
Cooper, E.B. and Rustin, L. (1985). Clinician attitudes toward stuttering in the United States and Great Britain: a cross-cultural study. *Journal of Fluency Disorders* 10, 1–17.
Cooper, E.B., Eggertson, S.A. and Galbraith, S.A. (1971). Clinician personality factors and effectiveness: a three study report. *Journal of Communication Disorders* 4, 40–43.
Dalton, P. and Hardcastle, W. (1990). *Disorders of Fluency*, 2nd edn. London: Whurr Publishers.
Dalton, P. and Dunnett, G. (1990). *A Psychology for Living*. London: Dunton Publishing.
Fransella, F. (1972). *Personal Change and Reconstruction*. London: Academic Press.
Gregory, H. (1978). *Controversies about Stuttering Therapy*. Baltimore, MD: University Park Press.
Hayhow, R. and Levy, C. (1989). *Working with Stuttering: A Personal Constuct Therapy Approach*. Oxfordshire: Winslow Press.
Haynes, W.O. and Oratio, A.R. (1978). A study of clients' perceptions of therapeutic effectiveness. *Journal of Speech & Hearing Disorders* 43, 21–33.

Kanfer, F.H. (1980). Self-management methods. In: Kanfer, F.H. et al. (Eds), *Helping People Change*. New York: Pergamon.

Lay, R. (1982). Stuttering: training the therapist. *Journal of Fluency Disorders* 7, 63–69.

Leahy, M.M. (1994). Attempting to ameliorate student therapists' negative stereotype of the stutterer. *European Journal of Disorders of Communication* 29(1), 39–49.

Murphy, A. and Fitzsimmons, R. (1960). *Stuttering and Personality Dynamics*. New York: Roland Press.

Schriberg, L.D., Bless, D.M., Carlson, K.A., Filley, F.S., Kwiatowski, J. and Smith, M.E. (1977). Personality characteristics, academic performance and clinical competence in communicative disorders majors. *Asha* 19, 311–321.

Sheehan, J.G. (1979). Current issues on stuttering and recovery. In: Gregory, H.H. (Ed.), *Controversies about Stuttering Therapy*. Baltimore, MD: University Park Press.

Stengelhofen, J. (1993). *Teaching Students in Clinical Settings*. London: Chapman & Hall.

St. Louis, K.O. and Lass, N.J. (1981). A survey of communicative disorders students' attitudes toward stuttering. *Journal of Fluency Disorders* 6, 49–80.

Van Riper, C. (1975). The stutterer's clinician. In: J. Eisenson(Ed.), *Stuttering: A Second Symposium*. New York: Harper & Row.

Wingate, M.E. (1988). *The Structure of Stuttering: A Psycholinguistic Analysis*. New York: Springer Verlag.

Woods, C.L. and Williams, D.E. (1976). Traits attributed to stuttering and normally fluent males. *Journal of Speech & Hearing Research* 19, 267–278.

Chapter 9
The Association for Stammerers and 'At the Receiving End': a Stammerer's View

NORBERT LIECKFELDT

In 1978, participants of an intensive course at the City Lit centre in London came together and, encouraged by their speech therapist Peggy Dalton, joined with an existing self-help group to form the Association for Stammerers (AFS). The idea was for stammerers to cooperate in order to create facilities to help them to cope better, particularly with fluency maintenance problems. The element of self-help was to remain the most important driving force behind AFS. Lately, another element has been coming into the equation: the recognition that helping others, by campaigning for better speech therapy provision, for example, or by offering advice to parents of stammering children, is just as much a facet of self-help, if not more so.

After 10 years, the Association had grown so much that it was decided to set up a national office and employ full-time staff. AFS has never looked back since. At present, it has the largest membership of any stammering organisation in Europe and is the second largest organisation of its kind worldwide. About 20% of its members are speech therapists. However, only adult stammerers have the right to vote, as it was felt that speech therapists have vested interests which might clash with those of the Association. Cooperation between the Association and the speech therapy profession is, however, very close. Currently, AFS's constitution is under review with the ultimate aim of giving parents the right to vote on behalf of their children, and of changing the Association's name. It receives the lion's share of its funding through donations from companies and charitable trusts, supplemented by grants from the Department of Health and self-generated income (membership subscriptions, book sales, individual donations etc).

The Association works mainly in the field of advice and information, and is operating a full service, receiving more than 2500 requests for information each year, by mail or telephone. Free information packs, tailored to the needs of adults, teenagers, children and parents, as well as speech therapists, are available and can be supplemented by additional information on many aspects of stammering therapy. The Association has compiled a directory of speech therapy provision in the United Kingdom, with information about speech therapy services in every health authority. We also list specialist services (where existing), as well as self-help groups, speech therapists working in private practice and intensive courses. This enables us to point every enquirer in the direction of his or her health therapy service, usually without the stammerer having to go through a general practitioner.

AFS operates a postal lending library where books and videos about stammering, as well as relaxation tapes, are available to members for the price of postage. As part of our service for speech therapists, the Association is planning to establish a video rental service based at the national office.

AFS's quarterly magazine *Speaking Out* is the main forum for discussion amongst stammerers in the United Kingdom, with articles on stammering therapy and research, letter pages, book and video reviews etc. It has a circulation of 2500 per issue and is held in high regard by stammerers, speech therapists and the international stammering community. AFS's sister organisations worldwide receive copies regularly, and an overseas subscription service for people overseas has been established.

One of the main problems faced by stammerers is the feeling of isolation. Before joining AFS, I had only ever met one other stammerer which is understandable because, with only 1% of the population stammering and many of us being very good at hiding the stammer, it is not easy to find us in a crowd. AFS is operating various schemes to help overcome this sense of isolation. Open Days are organised all over the country, where stammerers come together to discuss various topics of interest or just to meet and have a chat. The Association operates a telephone link scheme where stammerers exchange telephone numbers to encourage them to make more use of the telephone. Knowing that the person at the other end of the line also stammers makes this very much easier. The audiotape corresponding service works similarly, only here members exchange tapes on which they have recorded messages. There is also a pen-pal service.

During the last few years it has become more and more obvious that there was a great need for the concerns of stammering children and their parents to be taken into account. AFS tried to meet this by setting up the 'Helping Stammering Pupils Project' (HSPP) to facilitate the exchange of information between schools, pupils, teachers and parents. Not least because many adult stammerers have unpleasant memories of their school days, it was decided that this should be one of the main areas of AFS's work. At the moment, the HSPP has about 600 members comprising pupils, parents, teachers and speech therapists. This gives the Association access to a network of interested people which is probably unparalleled anywhere. AFS has held the first ever consultation meeting in London, where stammering pupils and their parents joined with teachers and therapists to discuss the problems stammerers are faced with at school: reading out in class, oral exams, bullying etc. This meeting was so successful that others quickly followed: in Sheffield and Glasgow in 1994. AFS commissioned research at Sheffield University's Department of Psychology, which resulted in an information pack on 'Bullying and the Dysfluent Child in Primary School' (available from AFS). The aim of this consultation process is to produce a comprehensive teachers' information pack which outlines workable solutions to the problems commonly encountered by stammering schoolchildren. A report will also be presented to the Department For Education.

In the past AFS has found that an ever-increasing number of the enquiries received have been concerned with the problems of children and the questions of their parents. To meet this demand AFS set up a Parents' Helpline, sponsored by British Telecom. Trained volunteers are available to advise parents on the best way of getting professional help for their children. Many parents also find it helpful to speak to others in the same position, so AFS is offering the services of the Parents' Network, where telephone numbers are swapped and parents can speak to each other, compare notes and exchange experiences.

It was only recently that AFS moved into the areas of research and campaigning. Initially, AFS limited itself to issuing, after consultation with its members, comments about various 'alternative' treatment methods, as practised by Andrew Bell, Dr Martin Schwartz, Dave McGuire *et al.* The first project was the setting up of a research database, basically a computerised bibliography of articles and monographs about stammering, listed under various headings. So anyone looking for information on, for example, a possible connection between epilepsy and stammering will be able to get references to a number of articles written about the subject.

AFS is cooperating with Dr Pam Enderby's Stammering Research Project at the Speech and Language Therapy Research Unit, Frenchay Hospital, Bristol. She is concerned with finding objective outcome measurements for stammering therapy, with the view of improving its value in the eyes of health care purchasers. This is important for stammerers as, without objective criteria on the outcome of therapy, we have no means by which to measure the expertise of the therapist.

AFS is currently applying to the Department of Health to fund a proposed 'Primary Healthcare Workers' Project', which would give information about the need for early treatment in stammering children, mainly to general practitioners and health visitors. This is important as our work on the Parents' Helpline has shown a lack of understanding of the importance of early intervention by the healthcare profession. This would be followed by measuring the effect of this information campaign on referral figures to speech therapy departments.

In 1993, after years of campaigning for better NHS stammering therapy, AFS entered a new phase of direct lobbying of health and other relevant authorities. The Association is making carefully considered representations in three types of situations: where an existing quality service is under threat; where a real opportunity for improvement exists; and where no service at all is being offered. In Glasgow, for example, the need for a specialist centre for the treatment of stammering in children has been put to the Health Board; AFS has written to the Home and Health Departments of the Scottish Office, urging financial support for a Scotland-wide service, and has sought support from Members of Parliament from all parties in Scotland.

AFS is in constant contact with other European stammering organisations through its membership of ELSA (the European League of Stammering Associations). ELSA's aim is to tap the diversity of views and experiences between the various countries for the benefit of all its constituent organisations.

For mainly linguistic reasons, however, AFS is cooperating most closely with the two American stuttering organisations, the National Stuttering Project (NSP) and the Speak Easy Foundation. The NSP is the largest stammering organisation worldwide. For information on these, please contact:

John Ahlbach
National Stuttering Project
2151 Irving Street
Suite No. 208
San Francisco
CA 94122-1609, USA
Tel: 415-566-5324

Bob Gathmann
The Speak Easy International Foundation Inc.
233 Concord Drive
Paramus
NJ 07652, USA
Tel: 201-262-0895.

There is also a unique organisation in the United States called the Speech Foundation of America. It produces a range of well-respected books and videos on stammering, which are distributed in the United Kingdom by AFS. The contact address is:

Speech Foundation of America
PO Box 11749

Memphis
TN 38111-0749, USA.

For any further information, please contact:

The Association for Stammerers
15 Old Ford Road
London E2 9PJ
Tel: 0181 983 1003; fax: 0181 983 3591.
Parents' Helpline: 0181 981 8818.

At The Receiving End: A Stammerer's View

Everything about stammering is very personal and highly individual. So
is this contribution. It is my view, my experience, the service I would like
to see – informed, however, by my work for the Association for Stammerers.

Many stammerers in the United Kingdom will have benefited greatly
from speech therapy – I am one of them. Others will never see a therapist, partly because they do not know such a service exists, or because
they do not wish to undergo therapy. Others feel perfectly happy with
their stammer and see no need for a change, or feel that speech therapy
would be the wrong approach for them. Amongst AFS's membership,
there are those whose lives have been transformed by therapy, others
where therapy has failed to show any success, as well as those who
regard speech therapy as, at best, useless, if not downright harmful. Why
is that?

The Problems

Under the regulations of the British National Health Service, stammering
is a recognised condition warranting treatment. Every health authority is
obliged to provide treatment, but only within budgetary constraints. The
drawbacks of this are obvious, especially with a National Health Service
in financial difficulties. Many health authorities use 'non-vital' services as
a financial buffer, to cut costs. After all, no one ever died of stammering!

This, then, is the first problem: some health authorities have reduced
their service. Sometimes this happens for a good reason, for example
when there is a very good specialist service in a neighbouring, easily
accessible location. More often than not, however, it is mere cost
cutting: sometimes, the adult service is cut altogether, and the child
service is so strained that the speech therapists cannot meet the treatment guidelines set down by the College of Speech and Language Therapists (for example, seeing a person presenting with the stammer within
eight weeks for an initial assessment). The fact is that there are some

areas in the country where speech therapy provision, especially for adults, is inadequate.

Most health authorities, however, do provide some sort of service for stammerers. These services usually operate on a self-referral basis, which is important for two reasons: many adult stammerers are too embarrassed by their condition to speak about it to their doctor. It might be that their stammer is exacerbated by speaking to someone 'in authority', as it were, or perhaps the stammer in itself is not very noticeable but causes severe psychological problems. Whatever the reasons, to be able to speak directly to someone who will understand the problem without lengthy explanations can be a great help. Then there are the parents of small children who are just developing a disfluency. They are very often told by a general practitioner or health visitor to ignore the stammer, that it will go away on its own. Neither the doctor nor the health visitor, however, has the professional knowledge to make this judgement: only a speech therapist can determine what is a normal phase of disfluency and what are the beginnings of a stammer. To insist, in the face of a doctor's opposition, on seeing a therapist is not easy and this problem is neatly sidestepped by being able to contact the speech therapy manager directly.

So, after finding the speech therapy contact, and after getting an appointment for an assessment, there is yet another problem: many speech therapists do not actually know very much about stammering and its treatment. This is understandable as (a) stammering constitutes only a very small part of most therapists' workload and (b) not very much is known about the causes of stammering. There is also not a great deal in the way of serious research into the long-term benefit of therapy. This absence of 'hard facts' can make a therapist's work frustrating. There tends to be a large gap between the client's expectations and the therapist's capabilities. Especially when dealing with adults, therapy often starts by having to tell the patient that there is no cure, that all the therapist can offer is ways of handling the stammer in a better way. This is a difficult concept for many stammerers to accept, but it probably does not do a lot for the therapist either.

So, in many cases, the stammerer will come across a speech therapist who will attempt to help by using a few choice methods, such as slowed speech, soft contact, block modification etc. Sometimes, little or no attention is paid to the needs and wishes of the stammerer, or to the fact that stammering, especially in adults, is not just a physiological condition. Renee Byrne, in her book *Let's Talk about Stammering*, uses Sheehan's excellent iceberg comparison in which, as with a real iceberg, the visible part of the stammer is usually only a small part of the problem. With some stammerers, what you hear is what you get – the audible stammer is the main problem, whereas psychological factors are not really an issue. This, however, is rare. With most stammerers, the stammer is only a small part of the problem; much more important are the feelings associated with the stammer. A therapy based on learning speech techniques (which is often all the non-specialist speech therapists can offer) is usually not sufficient, as the psychological aspects of stammering are not addressed.

When I started therapy, I was almost 30 years old. I knew my stammer like nobody else, and I knew what I wanted. I had the good fortune to see a specialist in stammering therapy, and after some initial hesitation I made it quite clear that I did not feel the need to become fluent through fluency techniques. Because my stammer is relatively mild, I had the luxury of being able to reject them. What I loathed about my stammer was not that it might make me sound ridiculous in certain situations, but that it sometimes denied me control over what I could or could not do at certain times. I wanted help to feel more in control, without breathing exercises or slowing my speech down. What I got out of it was the realisation that the stress of trying to hold on to this kind of control might not be very helpful when it comes to maintaining an acceptable degree of fluency. This, as I pointed out earlier, is a very personal experience: other stammerers will require other things from therapy. Although I reject fluency techniques, they might be just the thing a severe stammerer needs. What we need is a specialist who can lay out the options and let us choose.

But then, who is a specialist? There is, of course, the Specialist Interest Group in Disorders of Fluency (part of the College of Speech and Language Therapists). Membership of this group, however, is open to every speech therapist with an interest in stammering, and does not denote any specialist status. The College's definition of who is a specialist in the treatment of stammering is 'therapists [who] should have received postgraduate training and at least two years working with fluency disorders'. This, of course, neither defines the phrase postgraduate training nor does it tell us anything about how often the therapist sees a stammer in the prescribed two-year period. What is lacking are objective and generally recognised qualifications. The Association for Stammerers' official position is that it would like to see this remedied by the establishment of national centre(s) of excellence in the treatment of stammering. These, in my personal opinion, should not only be places of treatment but also sites for research: what we urgently require are objective criteria for the success of the various therapy approaches, especially when it comes to maintenance. It is very easy to make a stammerer fluent, but will it last? As long as we have no answer to this question, how can we make choices, how can we judge the quality of treatment and, in the final analysis, the quality of the therapists treating us? In the absence of these criteria, the centre(s) would serve as a training ground for therapists who want to specialise in the treatment of stammering. Only after a certain time at the centre, working with stammerers under the supervision of the experts, would they become specialists themselves.

This, then, is what I would ideally like to see: a speech therapy service sufficiently funded to be able to accommodate stammerers' needs; a specialist speech therapist in every health authority who deals with stammering; a wide variety of therapy methods on offer, with the choice being made in close consultation with the stammerer. Intensive courses are an excellent idea, but what many adult stammerers in a job would also need are provisions for speech therapy outside office hours. What I would like to see is an intensive educational campaign for doctors and health visitors, so that I no longer hear from parents of teenage stammerers who were told by their doctor 10 years ago to ignore the stammer. What I would like to see is for the therapists who have worked hard to make a difference to stammerers' lives to be given the opportunity, the training and the tools to become even more effective.

Index